Cancer and Creativity

> Works of art are indeed always products of having-been-in-danger, of having-gone-to-the-very-end in an experience, to where no one can go further. The further one goes, the more one's own, the more personal, the more unique an experience becomes, and the work of art, finally, is the necessary, irrepressible, most valid possible expression of this uniqueness.
>
> Rainer Maria Rilke, letter to Clara Rilke, June 24, 1907

Cancer and Creativity is a dialogue between accounts by cancer patients and survivors and a more clinical consideration and theoretical discussion from a psychoanalytic point of view of using creativity in coping with serious illness. The contributions featured demonstrate the power of creative expression as a tool for dealing with somatic, chronic and potentially life-threatening illnesses, giving patients a way of expressing and managing their individual cancer journeys and its attendant emotional sequelae.

Ten artist-patients and survivors, who were involved in several long-term art therapy groups, give accounts of their experiences with cancer and with their support group, where they create paintings, embroidery, digital photography, comic books, maps and other works to express their experiences of being diagnosed and treated for cancer. The contributors describe their symptoms and their relationships to physicians and family members in words and visual representations. The book also addresses the experience of the public when they are confronted with art by cancer patients. Dreifuss-Kattan's own work as a psychoanalyst and art therapist informs her approach to the art space as what Winnicott calls a "transitional space," influenced by both the personal psychological experience and the physical environment. Dreifuss-Kattan closes her discussion with a reflection on terminal cancer care and the complex transferential and countertransferential relationship between patient and therapist. The book ends with a practical guide for both therapy groups, as well as individuals at home, to creatively address their experiences with cancer and its treatments.

Cancer and Creativity will be of great interest to psychoanalysts, psychoanalytic psychotherapists, psychooncologists and art therapists, as well as health professionals working in oncology and in palliative care.

Esther Dreifuss-Kattan, PhD, is the president of the New Center for Psychoanalysis 2016–2018 in Los Angeles, a senior faculty member and a member of the Archival Committee, the Diversity Committee and Program Committee. Her previous book with Routledge was *Art and Mourning: The role of creativity in healing trauma and loss* (2016).

Cancer and Creativity
A Psychoanalytic Guide to
Therapeutic Transformation

Edited by Esther Dreifuss-Kattan

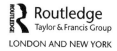
Routledge
Taylor & Francis Group

LONDON AND NEW YORK

First published 2019
by Routledge
2 Park Square, Milton Park, Abingdon, Oxon OX14 4RN

and by Routledge
711 Third Avenue, New York, NY 10017

Routledge is an imprint of the Taylor & Francis Group, an informa business

British Library Cataloguing-in-Publication Data
A catalogue record for this book is available from the British Library

Library of Congress Cataloging-in-Publication Data
Names: Dreifuss-Kattan, Esther, editor.
Title: Cancer and creativity: a psychoanalytic guide to
therapeutic transformation / edited by Esther-Dreifuss Kattan.
Description: Abingdon, Oxon; New York, NY: Routledge, 2019. |
Includes bibliographical references and index.
Identifiers: LCCN 2018030643 (print) | LCCN 2018033227 (ebook) |
ISBN 9781351206273 (Master) | ISBN 9781351206266 (Web PDF) |
ISBN 9781351206259 (ePub) | ISBN 9781351206242 (Mobipocket/Kindle) |
ISBN 9780815383253 (hardback: alk. paper) |
ISBN 9780815383260 (pbk.: alk. paper) | ISBN 9781351206273 (ebk)
Subjects: | MESH: Art Therapy | Neoplasms—psychology |
Psychotherapeutic Processes | Creativity
Classification: LCC RC489.A7 (ebook) | LCC RC489.A7 (print) |
NLM WM 450.5.A8 | DDC 616.89/1656—dc23
LC record available at https://lccn.loc.gov/2018030643

ISBN: 978-0-8153-8325-3 (hbk)
ISBN: 978-0-8153-8326-0 (pbk)
ISBN: 978-1-351-20627-3 (ebk)

Typeset in Times New Roman
by codeMantra

To my children and their children:

To my children Sarit and Jonathan with Sophie, Daniela, Max and Gabi and Pavel with Noemi

In loving memory of Zizi Raymond, Howard Bass, Chaya Spalter

and

my parents Max and Suzanne Dreifuss-Levy

Contents

Figures

Preface

It was a great honor and privilege to be invited to participate in the curatorial planning of the *From the Canvas to the Couch: Art and Cancer* exhibition held from April 14 through June 14, 2013, at the New Center for Psychoanalysis in Los Angeles that formed the basis for this book. *From the Canvas to the Couch* was a remarkable assembly of artworks by both trained and so-called outsider artists who have used their art making in response to medical adversity. This diverse group of artists was united only by their feminine gender and cancer diagnosis. The broad theme was "responding to cancer" while the specific artistic forms traverse the processes of photography, collage, drawings, embroidery, knitting sculpture and installation.

The success of the exhibition rested on the willingness of the artists to delve deeply into their psyche to discover the fit between their personal encounter with their specific experience with a potentially life-threatening illness and the creative process, materials and final form of their artistic production. The variety of artistic form and use of material lead to a richer and ultimately more nuanced viewer experience. The stories told were individual stories, but together the work demonstrated the process of art as a healing tool as an overarching theme. Through public presentation, the exhibition created a space for the artists to step away from their work and contemplate their output. The exhibition offered the artists, Christine Carey, Corrine Lightweaver, Ashley Myers-Turner, Zizi Raymond and Mary E. Walter, the chance to take charge. In earlier exhibitions at the Premiere Oncology Foundation, Howard Bass showed his amazing talent in which he mapped out his personal cancer journey with humor and sadness. And in the Healing Arts group at the Simms/Mann UCLA Center for Integrative Oncology, Loene Trubkin and Teresa O'Rourke expressed in their paintings their personal internal dialogue with cancer and its often overwhelming and frightening treatments.

They gifted family, friends and the community of professionals in oncology and in the healing arts with the prospect of connecting with the very private and personal experiences of a cancer patient. The panel discussion with the artists at the opening reception provided a venue for the celebration of the great accomplishment of this group of artists. It also helped viewers recognize that the process of making art affords us the opportunity to deal creatively with the exigencies of life itself and opens a venue to a deeper psychological insight, in order to work through the often traumatic experience of having cancer with its treatments.

—Suzanne Isken, Executive Director, Craft &
Folk Art Museum in Los Angeles

Acknowledgements

I am very grateful for the trust, confidence and generosity of each contributor who contributed in words and with their art to this collaborative, creative book. I realize that it is not easy to share such a private and personal journey with cancer with a wide audience. These journeys are often traumatic, but they can also bring forth unusually artistic expressions and joy.

This book would not have been possible were it not for the generosity of the Simms/Mann UCLA Center for Integrative Oncology and its executive director Anne Coscareli PhD, the Darcie Denkert Norton Director of Psychosocial Care and the Director of the Simms/Mann UCLA Center of Integrative Oncology, and Adjunct Professor the David Geffen School of Medicine. Anne allowed me to lead the *Healing Arts Group* for the last 16 years with her full support and with very little interference. Marcia Britvan is a very helpful administrator at the Simms Mann who offers kind support when I come to the center each Wednesday. Yasmin Elie not only prepares the art room for the weekly group meetings but also organizes my overflowing art materials cabinet in a kind and professional manner.

Most of the authors and artists of this book came out of the *Cancer and Creativity* group that was housed at the Premiere Oncology Foundation in Santa Monica, California, directed by Robbie Gluckson, who is now the Director of Marketing, Development and Community Outreach at the Department of Medicine UCLA Health. Her loving support for the patients who participated and her enthusiasm for art therapy were wonderful and made each Tuesday afternoon a pleasure in this large, beautiful art room. Her openness and support for putting up regular art exhibitions in their large lobby was encouraging and inspiring to the artists and myself and allowed us to create the best work possible.

I am grateful for the strong and warm reception and support of the two physicians of Premiere Oncology, Lee S. Rosen MD, Health Science Clinical Professor of Medicine Division Hematology and Oncology at the Ronald Reagan UCLA Medical Center and of Jonathan W. Goldman, MD Assistant Professor at UCLA Hematology and Oncology. Both of them were supportive and interested in our group, attended the receptions for our exhibitions and extended a warm welcome to the exhibiting artists and their family and friends. They were also welcoming to all our group members, cancer patients who are treated in different cancer centers around Los Angeles. Thanks to the generous support of their Premiere Foundation, the group was free for all patients

My thanks go to Randi Grossman, MPH, the Executive Director of Chai Lifeline, a national nonprofit organization that helps families with a child who has cancer. Randi's support in using art therapy for some of these children or their impacted siblings allowed me to get experience in the psychodynamic and art therapeutic realm with children and adolescents. Her empathy and steady interest in my art-based workshops with children and adolescents with cancer made this difficult work fun and interesting for the kids and resulted in less trauma and in great art exhibitions that illuminated the children's faces. We formed a good team together with Alyssa Wiesel, licensed Family and Marriage Therapist and Art Therapist at Chai Lifeline, putting on art-based workshops and art exhibitions for children and adolescents with cancer and their siblings who were all impacted by cancer trauma.

Many thanks go to Dr. Lonnie Zeltzer, Distinguished Professor of Pediatric Anesthesiology, Psychiatry and Biobehavioral Science and Director of the Pediatric Pain and Palliative Care Program of Pediatric Hematology-Oncology at the David Geffen School of Medicine at UCLA. Lonnie's expertize in treating chronic pain and in pediatric oncology and her support for art therapy for children with chronic pain was welcomed and she taught me very much.

The late Dr. Edith Kramer, Professor and founder of the Art Therapy Program at New York University and one of the founders of art therapy, guided me early on. Without our subsequent friendship, combined with her rich clinical insight into combining art therapy with psychodynamic psychotherapy, this book would not have happened. As my dissertation advisor many years ago, she not only supported me when I began working with cancer patients in the late 1970s but also supervised me much earlier in my first job as an art therapist at Chestnut Lodge. Her own art making inspired me to focus on my art as well, a continuing pleasurable and satisfying experience.

The late George Martz, MD, professor in Oncology, fostered my psychooncological approach to art therapy together with the late Fritz Meerwein, MD, Liaison Psychiatrist and Professor of Psychosomatic Medicine and Oncology and Psychoanalysis at the University Hospital in Zurich Switzerland. Their emphasis on research as well as psychoanalytic supervision gave my work depth and allowed me to understand my oncology patients much better through the art they created.

I would like to thank my friend Gabriele Schwab, Chancellor's Professor of Comparative Literature at the University of California, Irvine, and Research Psychoanalyst at the New Center for Psychoanalysis for reading my introduction and offering her insights and suggestions.

Mike Gales, MD, the program director at the New Center for Psychoanalysis, was always kind enough to allow me to present some of my thoughts and research at scientific meetings. I received feedback and encouragements from my colleagues at the New Center that made these chapters much better.

My colleague Laurie Wilson, PhD, Art Historian, Research Psychoanalyst and Art Therapist invited me to present at the American Psychoanalytic Meetings in New York City in the Art and Psychoanalysis group. The discussions that followed proved to be helpful and stimulating.

My friend Suzanne Isken, the Executive Director of the Los Angeles Craft Art and Folk Art Museum (CAFAM), and one of the authors in this book, was instrumental in putting on the exhibition *From the Canvas to the Couch* at the New Center for Psychoanalysis in Los Angeles. Her curatorial experience and insight into Outsider Art and the Arts and Crafts movement contributed to its success and to this consequent book.

My appreciation goes to my two editors who helped me with several drafts of each chapter, Gabriel Sessions, PhD from Philadelphia and Ben Garceau, PhD who lives in Irvine. Their insights, questions and suggestions for change, as well as their knowledge of the craft of editing contributed greatly to the project of this book.

Cecila Peck, the Executive Director of the New Center for Psychoanalysis was my rock. Without her focused help at the New Center for Psychoanalysis, I could not have had written this book and at the same time been the president of the New Center. She became a reliable force and an empathic friend. I am thankful that she understood how I tried to dance at several weddings at the same time and introduce change and new initiatives at the Center. Thank you!

Many thanks go to my good friends Lesley and Brian Kleinman and Michelle and Allan Willner and their families for their warmth, kindness and generosity. I would not have known what to do without them here in LA with my family so far away.

I would also like to thank Diana and Jed Buchwald, both distinguished Professors at the California Institute for Technology, for their friendship. They feel like family to me. Their scholarship and creative output shows me that with enough Sitzleder one can create amazing things.

Appreciation goes to Robert Ross, my former classmate at the Southern California Psychoanalytic Institute, and now trusted friend, for his presence, kindness and exellent insights.

Thanks to my good friend Karin Dreiding from Zurich for being such a generous friend for 57 years. Her support helped me to work on this book with more peace of mind. The fun vacation in NYC December 2017 helped us both to catch up on all of the arts. What can be better!

Thanks also to my brother Alex and sister-in-law Marlise for their kindness and for taking me to the Alps last year. The highlight was the Swiss architect Peter Zumthor's St. Benedict Chapel in the village of Sumvitg in Graubuenden. His play with the light of the sun and its shadows was inspiring, and sometimes I imagine myself sitting there again and hoping for creative inspiration.

The kind generosity of both my brother Walter and sister-in-law Claudette are humbling, and I could not have finished this book without their generous help and reliable, consistent friendship.

My creative and productive daughters, Sarit Kattan Gribetz, and Gabriela Khazanov Kattan, who both write and publish regularly in their respective fields, function as amazing role models for me. I am always amazed that they still come up with suggestions or edits for my work, in spite of families and full-time jobs. Together with their equally creative husbands, Jonathan Gribetz and Pavel Khazanov, who also write and publish, they inspire in their kindness and I appreciate their help, insights and patience for this book.

My grandchildren, Sophie, Daniela, Max and Noemi are the best. They make me smile and very happy be it on FaceTime or when visiting them on the East Coast or wherever they are in the world at a given time. Thank you!

Contributors

Esther Dreifuss-Kattan, PhD, ATR-CB Editor is a psychooncologist, art therapist, psychoanalyst and an artist. She is on the faculty and president of the New Center for Psychoanalysis in Los Angeles. Esther has worked for 36 years with cancer patients and survivors in University Hospitals in Los Angeles, Zurich and Tel-Aviv. She has lead the Healing Arts Group at the Simms Mann UCLA Center for Integrative Oncology since 2005. She is the author of three books: Prazis der Klinischen Kunst Therapy *(Practice of Clinical Art Therapy)* (Hans Huber Verlag 1988), *Cancer Stories: Creativity and self-repair* (Analytic Press 1990) and *Art and Mourning: The role of creativity in healing trauma and loss* (Routledge 2016).

Howard Bass was as creative in business as he was with his art. He designed and built commercial and residential properties in both New Jersey and in Aspen. He always drew and expressed himself with painting, collage and small sculptures while going through treatment for lymphoma. His memory and artwork live on with family and friends.

Christine Carey was born in England during one of the coldest winters on record. The river Thames froze over and Big Ben stopped the day she was born. She came to Los Angeles in 1977 and has been creating clothes and art most of her life. Her latest work was born out of her experience with breast cancer and now lives in Santa Barbara with her cat Kipper.

Suzanne Isken joined the Craft and Folk Art Museum as Executive Director in February, 2011, where she has shaped initiatives to educate audiences about contemporary craft and folk art and support the creation of new work. Her curatorial credits include Man-Made: Contemporary Male Quilters and Material as Metaphor. Previously she served as the Director of Education at The Museum of Contemporary Art, where she initiated a museum-based training program with the University of Southern California Medical School. She has also collaborated with the New Center for Psychoanalysis and other institutes to create public programs in conjunction with the exhibitions of the work of Lucian Freud, Louise

Bourgeois and art and feminism. Isken received an MSW degree from the University of Southern California in 1977.

Corinne Lightweaver is an editor and artist who, following two bouts of cancer, found solace and healing in art making. Her art exhibition catalog *In the Breast of Health: Healing from Cancer through Art*, with Esther Dreifuss-Kattan, documented much of her journey.

Ashley Myers-Turner is a photographer and writer. When diagnosed with a malignant brain tumor, she combined her technical photography skills with her Master's degree in Dance/Movement Therapy to create a self-portrait series illustrating her physical and emotional experience of cancer. Ashley continues to make her art in Los Angeles.

Teresa O'Rourke-Shapiro is a member of a large extended family. As an educational therapist and public school teacher, she loves to help her students sing, read, dance, write, garden and play with color. She attributes the success of her journey through stage four lymphoma and heart surgery to the UCLA Simms Mann Healing Through Art Group facilitated by Esther Dreifuss-Kattan.

Zizi Raymond MFA was an artist who was educated at UCLA and UC Davis as well as at Skowhegan School of Painting and Sculpture. She had eight solo exhibitions and participated in many group exhibitions within the United States. Her art is part of the collections at Bard College Center for Curatorial Studies Museum, The Berkeley Art Museum, Oakland Museum and the UC Davis Art Museum. She fought mightily with breast cancer with grace, humor and great creativity.

Devon Raymond earned her BFA from The Juilliard School and spent many years working as a professional actress before turning to screenwriting. More recently she has begun writing nonfiction and has completed her first book, a memoir about overcoming the aftereffects of childhood sexual abuse. Devon has studied extensively with the UCLA Extension Writers Program and has attended nonfiction workshops with the Community of Writers at Squaw Valley, the New York State Writers Institute at Skidmore College and the Martha's Vineyard Writers Residency.

Loene Trubkin was a business leader and novice lawyer until cancer treatment made it impossible for her to continue in those professions. Since retiring, she has begun gardening, writing prose and poetry and painting. She lives in Los Angeles.

Mary E. Walter is a visual effects editor in the movie business, as well as a freelance cartoonist and illustrator. She is working toward completing her first graphic novel, *My Years in Track Pants*, inspired by her cancer journey with melanoma. She lives in Los Angeles.

Alyssa Wiesel, LMFT, ATR received her Bachelor's Degree at Columbia University and Master's Degree at Loyola Marymount University. Alyssa currently serves as the Director of Clinical and Community Programs at Chai Lifeline, a nonprofit organization that helps families who have a child with cancer, where she has worked for the last decade. Additionally, Alyssa has her own private therapy practice in West Los Angeles, specializing in work with children. She is also an artist and resides in Los Angeles with her husband and four children.

Introduction

Esther Dreifuss-Kattan

Artist: Teresa O'Rourke

In the early 1970s, I spent several years working as an art therapist at Chestnut Lodge, a psychoanalytic psychiatric hospital in Rockville, Maryland. There, I used art therapy to help patients understand their internal worlds, gain self-confidence and overcome their challenges. Visual expression often became a gateway for my patients to find words to express emotions and fears that paralyzed them. Art offered potential avenues for more holistic forms of healing that complemented traditional psychiatry and integrated therapeutic processes.

One day, when I came home from a long day at the hospital, I received a letter in the mail from an old friend, Myra. Myra and I had attended art school together in Switzerland. She wrote to tell me that, unfortunately, she had been diagnosed with Leukemia. She had just undergone one of the first bone marrow transplantations in Europe. In her letter, she confided in me that she wished that she had a forum in which to continue creating art. She explained how helpful it would have been for her to draw or paint during the weeks she spent in her hospital room in total isolation following her transplant.

Myra was searching for a creative way to process her cancer treatment. In the face of invasive medical procedures, pain and a daunting future, Myra felt lost, overwhelmed and sad. I realized that the methods of art therapy that I had been using at the psychiatric hospital could be adapted to help cancer patients like Myra, who confronted physical and psychological challenges because of cancer.

Myra's letter inspired me to leave Maryland and return to Switzerland. There, together with a team of oncologists, psychiatrists and psychoanalysts, I began developing art therapy methods and treatments specifically designed for those battling cancer. In my role as a medial art therapist, I saw both inpatient and outpatients at the oncology department in the University Hospital in Zurich. I worked with patients with tumors as well as those with systemic cancers, creating art and helping them work through their traumas.

For the last 40 years, I have devoted my professional career as an art therapist, psychoonchologist and psychoanalyst to helping cancer patients and survivors as well as their relatives, caregivers and medical professionals, through art and art therapy. This book grew out of my experiences working in hospitals, nonprofit organizations and in private practice. For almost two decades, I have facilitated the *Healing Arts Group* at the Simms/Mann Center for Integrative Oncology at the University of California in Los Angeles, and for several years I also led the *Cancer and Creativity Group* at the Premiere Oncology Foundation in Santa Monica. I also designed art-based therapy workshops for children and teenagers with cancer through a national nonprofit organization called Chai Lifeline.

Cancer and Creativity: A guide to therapeutic transformation emerged out of an art therapy group that met for four consecutive years at the Premiere Oncology Foundation. It features the art and reflections of seven Los Angeles artist-patients, along with a chapter focused on the art and words of children and teenagers. Through their art and essays, they demonstrate that visual art is a powerful tool for working through the multiple losses that occur when one faces cancer diagnoses and treatment. Their imaginative pieces take the form of installations, digital photography, collages, acrylic painting, embroidery, comic strip illustrations, cancer maps and superhero self-portraits. These powerful pictorial narratives and aesthetic practices explore the impact of trauma, loss, mourning and pain. They also display hope, strength and perseverance, which are part of every individual cancer journey.

Cancer and Creativity demonstrates the empowering and therapeutic role that creativity and artistic expression can play when battling cancer and when dealing with one's survival in the years thereafter.

Each essay in this book demonstrates a different way in which visual art can serve as a powerful tool to address and work through questions about personal identity, family relationships, anxiety about the future and fear of death and dying. All these complicated emotions are normal reactions to cancer diagnosis and can be worked through in imaginative and creative ways. Art making allows cancer patients and survivors to understand their bodies as well as their psyche, change their perceptions of illness and health and creatively address their cancer traumas.

Confronting diagnosis and the role of art therapy in navigating a world of illness

In an interview with Lauren Sedofsky, the French philosopher Alain Badiou discusses the concept of the emergence of the *New* (Sedofsky, 1994). The *New*—an unexpected and important situation that can come suddenly without warning, cannot be known from the onset, and seems rather random—requires active participation of one's personal agency. Being diagnosed with cancer can be considered such an event, a confrontation with the *New*, a situation that disrupts the status quo as a patient questions the value of truth that is initially challenging to accept and understand. A cancer diagnosis forces each person to activate his or her personal agency in a new and unfamiliar manner, as each particular cancer is unpredictable. The newly diagnosed patient, confronted with the *New*, is suddenly forced to acknowledge the multiplicity of these many new events, unfamiliar experiences, unknown times and the lack of control over one's schedule, health and future.

The *New* and its consequent events are both medically and emotionally complex and overwhelming. When a patient is first diagnosed with cancer, he or she is suddenly confronted with questions of infinity and finitude, as cancer triggers fears of death and dying. Patients question their identities: are they the same, different or other? Patients also try to find the right language for disturbing new emotions they had not necessarily previously experienced, including fear, sadness, grief, anger and depression. In addition to such existential questions, newly diagnosed patients are torn away from their familiar tongues as a novel language of cancer is forced upon them. They are suddenly inundated with multiple information streams related to a frightening world of cancer that they often have to strain to comprehend. There are confusing new situations and terminologies that accompany medication, chemotherapy protocols, blood tests, radiology interventions, surgeries, reconstructions, immunotherapy, innovative experimental trials, dietary requirements and hospice care. A newly diagnosed person with cancer must learn to read between the lines and listen to what doctors and nurses explain, which can itself cause anxiety and shame when a patient cannot understand or remember the details of these meetings. They also need to sort out the roles of various health workers within a medical hierarchy. As patients become dependent on this complicated, multilayered medical system for support, relief and healing, they find themselves grappling with these new overwhelming realities associated with illness and the medical world. Cancer patients realize that cancer will forever belong to their personal histories and will affect their relationships in the broader world. Initially cancer can be all encompassing and can overshadow one's entire life as well as the lives of others, including family and friends. While it can be overwhelming and at times confusing, with support and guidance patients can also gain control of their emotional relationship to their illness and create meaning from it.

Cancer is one of the most common, potentially life-threatening illnesses that can affect anyone at any time, any age and in any place. Over the years, cancer treatments have improved greatly and what was once a death sentence has become, often, a chronic or even a temporary illness. Traumatic responses to surgeries, reconstruction, aggressive chemotherapies, radiation therapy, small molecular targeted therapy, immunotherapy hormonal therapy and bone or stem cell transplantation can take place over many months or even years. While these medical treatments often cure patients of their cancer, they often also cause long-term physical reactions, acute fear, anxiety, depression and post-traumatic stress. Cancer support groups are important as part of an integrative approach to illness, and their efficacy has been demonstrated by recent research. Patients who attend these support groups are less depressed, more socially and physically active and might even live longer because they are happier. Art therapy and art making are two of the more established and effective integrative treatments for adults, teenagers and children who face cancer.

In a 2008 article entitled "Education of Creative Art Therapy to Cancer Patients: Evaluation and Effect," Visser and Hoog reported that 35 cancer patients (most of whom had breast cancer) took part in an exploratory evaluation to see if a class on Cancer and Creativity would help them better cope with cancer (Visser & Hoog, 2008). While patients reported disappointment that the class was too short, they were clear in follow-up discussions that the group had greatly improved their abilities to cope with their emotions, had awakened a renewed feeling of "conscious living" and that they felt an improvement in their creativity and quality of life. Another article, published in the journal *Psycooncology* by Wood, Molassiotis and Payne in 2012, compared research articles on the use of art therapy in the management of psychological symptoms for cancer patients. After analyzing 12 studies, they concluded that art therapy is successful as a psychotherapeutic approach. It addresses symptoms such as pain, facilitates the exploration of emotions related to loss, changes patients' sense of uncertainty, distracts them from worrying and facilitates mental well-being. Patients also reported that the nonverbal, embodied, aesthetic aspect of art therapy provides a distinctive addition to more traditional verbal psychosocial support in which they had also participated (Wood, Malassiotis, & Payne, 2011).

Art making in the context of a new and overwhelming situation such as a cancer diagnosis is so effective because it lifts a person out of their sense powerlessness and away from the "medical gaze" (Foucault, 1973, p. 145), far from the immanence of one's medical and psychological condition. As Foucault writes in *The Birth of the Clinic*, [the patient] "now requires to be the object of the gaze, indeed, a relative object, since what is being deciphered in him was seen as contributing to better knowledge of others" (Foucault, 1973, p. 83). Art can counterbalance the objectification of a patient within a medical milieu and return their agency and sense of self to them.

The positive effects of art therapy are best illustrated through a brief example. While today's medical staff try to communicate openly with their patients and are increasingly more mindful of engaging with their patients as whole people, many doctors still view a person's body as separate from their personal identity or psyche. The scientific narrative often overpowers the personal one as a patient is not seen or acknowledged in that moment in his singularity by an overworked medical team and by oncologists who, for their own self-preservation, often stay distant from their patients and prefer to relate to them in a collective sort of way (e.g., the 'breast cancer patient,' or the 'colon cancer patient' or the 'metastatic melanoma cancer patient') rather than becoming emotionally invested in each patient. Doctors who are tasked with caring for patients' physical needs thus often forget or do not have the time to inquire after the patient's emotional state, family relationships, professional affiliations and financial situation, which can leave patients feeling perplexed and anxious, as though they have not been fully seen. In Chapter 8, for example, Mary discusses how she was sent by her regular oncologist to another oncologist for nerve pain several months after her melanoma surgery. The doctor was annoyed to see her, as he felt there was no need for his service as the pain could not be treated, and she found him to be withdrawn and unpleasant. As a patient, she felt unseen and uncared for. In order to cope with her feelings of rejection and frustration, she created a collage out of colored papers that she titled *Stage 1 Melanoma? "Oh That's Easy."* In the piece, a small doctor looks down at the floor, rather than at her face, while she portrays herself with a huge red fuming head; inside of her brain she depicts a small figure representing herself crying as a little lake filled with tears begins to form, and yellow spikes of anger spark out of her mouth. A viewer of this piece can so clearly see that Mary was fuming at the perceived lack of empathy she experiences from her doctor, who responded to her pain as simply a nuisance since she only had stage I melanoma. Mary was initially taken aback by how strongly she represented her feelings, which made her realize how angry she was at the doctor even though she had stayed calm and polite in the examining room. Producing this work of art helped Mary to express—and eventually distance herself from—her feelings and to move on.

Spending time in hospitals or outpatient clinics, in the company of different healthcare workers and subjected to complicated treatments for long hours can be anxiety producing for the cancer patients. A wish can surface to replenish this threatening void with creative expression in order to counteract feelings of fragmentation, emotional confusion and the sense of emptiness created by fear and trauma. Art, with its aesthetic forms, can transcend time and can reframe the present, imbuing it with sacred meaning. Artistic expression allows us to counteract the notion of illness with psychological insight, and psychic fragmentation with psychic integration, resulting in the pleasure of expression through creative means. The artist is encouraged to inhabit the spaces she likes and the role she chooses to assume, within the parameters of her imagination and the creative space of the art studio. Imagination offers patients an escape to the world of colors and shapes, allowing them to recover their sense of self and personal agency after the cancer diagnosis, and some familiarity with one's personal treatments is achieved. Because each cancer and each patient is unique, each patient-artist is able to become their own creative individual, defined through their relationships to others as well as to their new medical context, and is empowered to organize these new encounters and experiences in visual and creative ways.

After a car accident, Teresa O'Rourke had an MRI to see if she was hurt. A tumor was discovered and she was sent to an oncologist, who diagnosed her with Lymphoma. After months of chemotherapy she was in remission for a short time and then relapsed and was urged to go through stem cell transplantation. They took cells by drawing her blood, then cleaned the blood cells up and later reinjected them into her veins. Teresa spent a couple of weeks in the hospital in a very sterile environment and then went back home. Soon thereafter, the doctors realized that she had developed an infection and would have to return to the hospital. Teresa is a trooper: she sees the positive side of things. But it took a full year to attain a full recovery.

Now Teresa feels much better. She is helpful to many of her family members and friends, as well as to her students with special needs. Her father passed away last year, and she travels frequently to Chicago to visit her aging mother who suffers from dementia. When she came back from one trip, she shared with the group members how she organized her mother's paintings and encouraged her to draw while she was there. She became an art therapist. When she came back to the Healing Arts group she made the following image (Figure I.1).

We see the white outline of a person in a white cloth with a pink head without facial features, and a baby wrapped up in a dark blue-black cloth; like the mother, only a pink face is visible without facial features. The background is brown and dark green. This painting was very moving to me. On the same trip to help with her mother's art, Teresa's niece had a first baby without much psychological support, and Teresa stepped in to help. This painting illustrated not only the niece with her new baby, but also I believe Teresa's own mother, who had regressed to a virtual baby. She is now taken care of by her daughter Teresa, who not long ago was severely physically regressed herself.

A third variation I recognized in this painting is that Teresa, now stronger after recovery from a couple of years of intensive cancer treatments, allowed herself to be taken care of as a helpless, regressed baby. This was only possible in retrospect. I, as her therapist, can now become the mother in the transference, allowing Teresa to safely regress in her art without falling apart in the outside world.

Artistic expression fueled by unconscious memory and association helps each patient to become self-aware, to think and to act in a determinable way, guiding the patient to their own creative response (Wacquant, 2005, p. 316). Expression through art allows the person with cancer to embody their feelings and their experience of loss and mourning. This creative

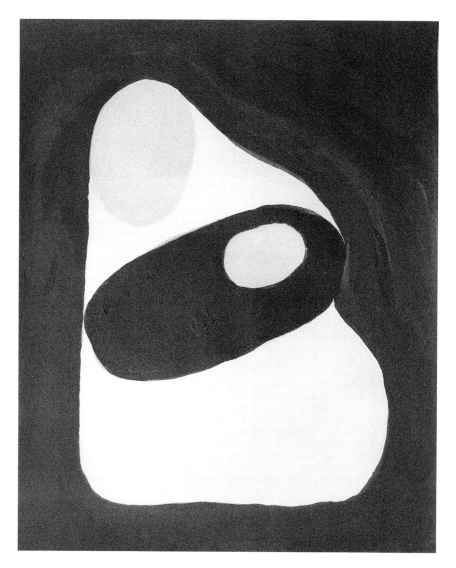

Figure I.I Teresa O'Rourke, "Mother and Infant," 2018, Acrylic Paint.

embodiment helps patient to 'inscribe' their memories, translate their feelings into signs and symbols and bring them from the inside out, projected onto the clay, canvas, fabric or onto a piece of paper. When feelings and experiences can be exteriorized and projected onto a canvas or sculpture, they can more easily and fruitfully be named, understood and addressed therapeutically.

Psychoanalytic frameworks for medical art therapy

My clinical experience has taught me that art making can enhance physical, emotional and social well-being, while identifying new meaning for the life not lived yet. Invention and exploration through art offers a creative way to become aware of different and difficult new emotional states and a place to explore them. Strong affects related to medical trauma such as fear, depression, anxiety and confusion are excellent triggers for exploration. Bereavement often triggers the imagination, tapping one's visual archive and resolidifying the cohesion of the self that becomes fragmented by fears of breakdown and of the unknown. The knowledge of the finitude of our lives and bodies not only brings forth loss and mourning but can also give rise to transformation and idealization, paving the way for externalizing feelings and ideas and fostering psychic representations into new imagery. Painting, drawing and making collages or embroidery can reinvigorate a capacity to mentalize, the imaginative mental activity that allows us to emotionally connect to needs, desires and feelings interrupted by the physical trauma of cancer. It calls for a creative wish to make connections, to link up to forgotten psychic representations and to fortify a new creative future together with loved ones, however short or long this future time might be. Through the creative reattachment with the good internalized object, be it a loving parent from the present or past, the therapist in the transference, a spouse, a child, other group members or with one's own creative force, a new future can be reimagined, despite a potentially life-threatening disease. This process engenders new hope and, ideally, renewed joy for life.

D.W. Winnicott, the English pediatrician and psychoanalyst, coined the term "transitional space," which he identified as the protective yet fluid space that forms between an infant and her parent. In *Subjects without Selves*, Gabriele Schwab discusses the transitional space as a space in which our imagination can bloom and where the relationship between an infant and her significant other can develop intersubjectively. In this transitional space of experience, a little child can find her first symbolic object, such as a blanket or toy, that helps the child mediate between conscious and unconscious experiences (Schwab, 1994). The transitional space of an art studio can function similarly to the supportive creative space between parent and child identified by Winnicott. It is a space in which an artist develops aesthetic forms through unconscious play and conscious elaborations.

The Philosopher Susan Langer writes that "Art is the creation of forms symbolic of human feelings" (Langer, 1953, p. 40). Langer constitutes the link to D.W. Winnicott and his theory of the transitional object. She suggested that it is the mother or father that allows for the primary creativity of the infant and that thus makes it possible for the baby to find and then imbue a toy or blanket with her own strong feelings, which Winnicott called the transitional object (Winnicott, 1971). This creative transitional object is "not me" but made mine, which allows a child to address subjects and boundaries and thereby facilitates a temporal separation from one's mother, father or caretaker. The transitional object helps the infant to make boundaries between Self and Other, between Me and Not-Me, inner and outer reality, conscious and not conscious, inviting dialogue and intersubjectivity through symbolization. Initially the infant has little differentiation, but can experience herself only through the parents' touch and looks, a recognition of a sort of a mirror structure through her body and touch (Schwab, 1994).

The art historian Ehrenzweig developed a theory about how people create aesthetic forms and how they are received by others (Ehrenzweig, 1967). Through a process of "unconscious scanning," an artist can come up with an idea, which they can then elaborate upon with conscious thoughts, symbols, forms and colors. The art that results can then facilitate insightful communication and interpretation that was not possible before. Sharing free associations about one's work with others, for example, can help the artist with cancer to slowly understand the layered content of his or her image on a deeper level. Through this process, unconscious and conscious themes surface and can be discussed and analyzed (Schwab, 1994).

Lacan argued that selfhood can only be accomplished with an outside object, be it the mother, the father or the mirror. He recognized the unconscious as being structured like a language and emphasized the symbolic structural signifier that emerges from our dynamic unconscious. He suggested that the visual of the *Imaginary* is brought forth by the early Mirror Stage of the infant. The mirror is first provided by parents through the infant's body which looks at and touches the mother/father and thus cultivates a body ego. The 'real' mirror helps to differentiate the image of the body from the image of the self. The infant recognizes in the mirror that her body is a bound and organized unit, a Gestalt of sorts that is really an illusion, but that fosters a desire for independence, in spite of present lack of skills, coordination and formation of boundaries (Schwab, 1994).

As we will see in Chapter 7, Ashley, a brain cancer survivor, was able to keep self-experience and self-image in harmony through an artistic photography project in which she created a series of digital self-portrait collages. Using the imaginary, Ashley was able to tap into her repressed disconcerting bodily perceptions in order to counteract her fears of fragmentation and disintegration. Her self-portrait photographs stabilized as well as destabilized her boundaries, as elements of self-estrangement surfaced due to disturbing symptoms. Externalizing her inner perception with the help of digital photography is not dissimilar to that of a mirror, as the projection from the actual mirror onto the photograph helps the patient to find a new Gestalt of herself at the time of physical and psychological fragmentation. Ashley photographed herself looking into the mirror, while overlaying her forehead that had harbored her brain cancer with her digital brain scan from the hospital. She attempted to relocate and find herself in the mirror after experiencing frightening seizures and unusual smells and delusions. The artist found herself in the mirror with a changed physicality and a new identity, but one that was not perceived as different by others. Looking at the finished product of her digital photo collages, she faced herself as though looking at the mirror. But the self that looked back at her was not her lost self but rather a newly integrated and healthy artist self. Similar to the very young child who recognized herself as a 'whole' person for the first time in the mirror, Ashley used artistic form and technology to recover and reassemble the pieces of her fragmented self due to brain cancer, and in the process reinvented herself and repaired—physically and emotionally— what had been lost or destroyed because of her cancer.

Through art making, this artist become aware of her own affective, reflective and resonating traumatic feelings and was able reestablish a link to her internal good objects and her internal life and eventually recovered her integrated imaginary self that then could be shared and regulated, counteracting the sense of a fragmented body. Making her digital collages allowed this artist to project a new sense of physical and psychological coherence (Lacan, 1977). This is but one important example of how artistic practices can become powerful tools that, through pictorial or abstract expressions can change one's perception of illness and health, life and death. Just as the mirror helps a baby to identify with her internal sense of self as well as with the external image of being separate between "I" and "You," the aesthetic dialogue with one's self can be initiated.

When one is confronted with trauma, expression through art can counteract the annihilation of one's internal "other," the primary empathic bond that often occurs as a result of traumatic experiences (Laub & Podell, 1995). Through the creative reattachment with the good internalized object, a loving parent from the present or past, or the therapist in the transference, art can bring forth a new order or organization and thus mute the traumatic haunting of fragmented memories. Aesthetic practices can reestablish a creative and verbal narrative and reestablish new connections, counteracting the disintegration and allowing the void associated with personal trauma to be filled up with creative works. The patient can deepen the emotional experience and imbue it with significance as it is contained in a safe framework (Laub & Podell, 1995).

One of the reasons that the art therapy groups that I lead with cancer patients work so effectively is because of the creative environment that we foster together. It is precisely within the creative space of the art studio that artists with cancer can feel simultaneously supported and free together with fellow cancer travelers. Being creative in the safe environment of the studio and contained within the group, the artists in the group can become a witness of their own and others' suffering, as they get more access to inner imagery that had been stored in their unconscious memory, now projected unto the canvas or a piece of paper. The sculpture or drawing that the trauma had brought forth can fill up this absence or void with ideas and forms that express human feelings and allow for a dialogue in their presence. The group members become empathic witnesses and hear and see in the pictures the reality of the very personal, individual cancer trauma (Laub & Podell, 1995). Having worked through the trauma creatively allows the cancer patient to reimagine a future in spite of a potentially life-threatening illness, engendering new hope and ideally a renewed joy of life.

Expression through art allows the person with cancer to embody their idea, feeling and experience of cancer into a concrete form through their art. This creative embodiment helps a patient to 'inscribe' their memories, to translate their feelings into colors, forms and symbols. Artistic work is very significant, as each of us knows that even the most ancient art and most modern art can touch us emotionally in the present. In trying to understand the creation of a piece of art, we can use the forming of our nightly dreams as a partial template. Unconscious fragments in a dream can turn into sensory perceptions that can then be transformed, when awake, into more cohesive symbols through conscious associations, informing both content and form. Dreams surfacing from the unconscious reconnect parts of our conscious awareness that have been severed through illness and loss. The creative, reparative functions of art making attempts a rapprochement with the external "healthy" mind and body perception, a new and different way to look at the world. We invite uncertainty that allows for new creative processes, openness, surprise and play. It is indeed the artistic form that integrates the experiences of illness, loss and trauma, fostering developmental and creative growth.

Experimentation in art means transgressing boundaries and inviting transitions that evoke new ideas and locate artistic forms that communicate personal aesthetic narratives about one's individual cancer journey in a given time framework. Fostering group discussions enhances psychological insight, artistic confidence and support and can aid in identifying the development of a new, healthier identity and a stronger sense of self in spite of cancer and its threat to one's physical integrity. Each patient's personal history and cancer experiences can change through access and insights from one's personal pictorial archive stored in our unconscious with its associations. The response of other group participants invites free association and openness, while offering comfort and empathy for each other, all sharing this sense of uncertainty with its fears and hope, embracing the capacity to listen and view creative surprise and insight.

Externalizing one's inner life through artistic activity helps in problem-solving, as the artist becomes aware of her affective, reflective and resonating communications with her loved ones, the group members and internal objects. It is one way to take control of the cancer patient's fate, change the perception of illness and health and address the trauma and its unconscious aspects. Creating aesthetic, subjective forms that can reach both inward and outward provokes meaningful discourse. Art is continuous and permanent and can at times be experienced as revolutionary—as a form of protest.

The philosopher Merleau-Ponty describes in his book "Eye and Mind" (1964) that the eyes are not only designated for seeing, but the entire body becomes a medium for seeing and being seen, as the body is a sensory object that can be sensed. Thus we can become particularly self-conscious when our body is not functioning well, even though that might not be perceived or noticed by anybody else. This sense complicates our relationship to our body and with the Other. An illness like cancer might make it necessary to reframe the discussion with ourselves, to view and feel our physical body as being seen from the outside, or in a painting from a distance in the realm of the imaginary, as Merleau-Ponty describes:

> My field of perception is constantly filled with a play of colors, noises and fleeting tactile sensations which I cannot relate precisely to the context of my clearly perceived world, yet which I nevertheless immediately 'place' in the world without ever confusing them with my daydreams.
> (Merleau-Ponty, 1945 [1962], p. xi)

In this creative world we can reimagine our body in a creative mindset and be empowered by our imagination and sensations as well as by our fragmented memory due to the cancer experience.

Bohleber, in his paper on the "Geography of the mind," refers to the mind's geography in metaphorical terms, as a place where our fantasies try to organize our psychic reality (Bohleber, 2011, p. 285). Sometimes these fantasies seem to be barely structured and are even chaotic, particularly after a trauma like a cancer diagnosis. At other times they might be well organized and can be presented through symbols and structures. This is a sign for Bohleber that the patient has recovered her inner personal and creative balance and can again communicate it to his or her psychoanalyst and art therapist. He suggests that these mental experiences often lie on a continuum and cannot really be fully classified. Verbal and artistic expressions can at times be both regressed as well as highly defined. Traumatic experiences often cannot be verbally expressed, but might more easily be communicated symbolically through artistic expression and the imaginary. Creative communications thus also help the psychoanalyst and art therapist to recognize internal states even without any words, for the therapist can catch a glimpse into a patient's psychic organization simply by viewing and analyzing a painting or a sculpture. In addition, art functions as a container to hold these confusing, often fragmented traumatic experiences for as long as needed, until the patient is ready to grapple with its content. Bohleber calls this new unconscious a "generative or relational unconscious" (Bohleber, 2011, p. 288).

Each of the artist-patients and survivors in this book who share their art and stories reacted differently to their cancer diagnosis and treatments, but they all use personal pictorial expression with different art materials and art forms to absorb or metabolize their trauma caused by cancer and its treatments. To work through mourning, creative reparation using any art modality helps us to reestablish our impacted psychological equilibrium. The artist with cancer often mourns not only present losses initiated by the cancer diagnosis and its treatments, but at the same time she or he address and revisits older losses from the past, preserved in their unconscious. Aesthetic, expressive and formal abilities allow these artist-patients to reconstruct their emotional experience in visual form in an attempt to connect to their selves as well as to the Other, the viewer. Giving creative form through our visualization and our imagination can stabilize our badly damaged self and reestablish the narcissistic balance that had become overwhelmed by archaic affects and fragmentation as a result of a potentially life-threatening illness with its intrusive, often aggressive treatments and fear of death.

Art making—with its symbolization and exteriorization at a time of personal loss and trauma that has been pushed into the psychic background—allows for a gradual modulation of affects. It also can initiate a personal reinvention by reconstructing one's past life and experiences and allowing an artist to become a witness of their own individualized journey with cancer. If there is no integration through artistic expression or with the help of a working through process in another form, no idealization can occur, but rather a depletion of the self takes place that can generate depression as well as despair. By expressing one's own story in images and symbols, the artist and cancer survivor demonstrates a wish to survive these losses and to take some distance from the cancer experience. Looking at one's own creation from a distance, outside of oneself, and at the same time sharing it with others who went through similar experiences, allows the cancer patient's personal internal and external witness to become stronger, fostering empathy, insight and more security. This newly expressed narrative in an innovative and artistic form can be substituted for the actual trauma that was brought forth by the cancer diagnosis and or its treatments, helping to regain cohesiveness and integration of the self. Creative expression can transcend the past and can become linked to the present in an attempt to gain balance and live with a less threatening future.

The talented artists featured in this book are mostly cancer survivors who were able to fill the void in the imaginary that was left by their cancer trauma because of surgeries, aggressive chemotherapies radiation, and multiple other medical interventions. Loss, bereavement and absence trigger their imagination, allowing their affects to be expressed through different artistic disciplines, and thus to help resolidify the cohesion of the self. The work of mourning through creative means leads to a new reality, a wish to continue living in order to create something in the present but of the past. As Joan Copjec has written, "The valorization of the creative act can create a new link between immortality and a sense of infinity, reestablishing in a sense and a feeling of permanence" (Copjec, 2002, p. 20). Through the reattachment with the internalized good object, a person from the past, or one's creative force, a future can be reimagined, in spite of a potentially life-threatening disease, engendering hope and even a joy of life.

Outline of the book

Chapter 1, *Sigmund Freud's Consultation Room and the Art Studio*, addresses the importance of providing a personal and safe consultation room and art studio environment. A safe space is a necessary starting point for the creation of art, especially among those facing illness. Such a safe space also fosters the ability to transcend bodily and physical concerns in order for artist-patients to enter into a dialogue with the imaginary and with hidden ideas and expectations. By introducing Freud's iconic consultation room, with its famous couch and his collection of antiquities and their personal meaning, this creative room becomes a transitional space for sharing sensitive personal memories and experiences. Analyzing Freud's sanctuary creates a segue to the contemporary art studio, which promises creative interchange between the art-psychotherapist and patient. This chapter also explores the idea of a space between the individual and the environment— the *"the potential space"*—that negotiates the boundaries between the self and the world and between subjectivity and culture, as it is theorized by D.W. Winnicott.

Chapter 2, *Art as a Transformational Object*, explores three intertwined relationships created in the process of art therapy with cancer patients: (1) the relationship between the physical symptoms of illness and the unconscious fears and emotions that these medical conditions evoke, (2) the relationship between art and its interpretation and (3) the relationship between patient-artists, who produce the art, and art therapists, who help them to understand its significance. The chapter also explores the meaning of artistic expression for the cancer patient, both psychologically and personally, and the way in which art embodies personal experience and brings forth and transmits affects that can be shared within the group process. The chapter centers on the close analysis of three small sculptures and one fabric mural created by the late Los Angeles artist and cancer patient Zizi Raymond. In our group sessions, Raymond described how she used these painted landscapes to visually describe her physical symptoms. Another member of the group, however, also helped Raymond to understand that, through these landscapes, she had also depicted her inner world and the internal symptoms that her cancer had produced but that had been more challenging to access. While initially such pictorial expressions might bring forth some anxiety both in the patient and therapist (as well as in other group members), with time everyone learns how mood, ideas and attitudes surface and can be understood. The chapter draws on Wilfred Bion's idea of what is "beyond memory and desire," in which memory surfaces out of the darkness and formlessness of the unconscious. This idea is applied to processes that the art-psychotherapist uses in order to approach each session with an open mind and helps the patient draw out memories and thoughts from their present state of mind.

Chapter 3, *One In Eight*, addresses the fact that one in eight women in the United States is diagnosed with breast cancer. With today's improved treatment methods and increased knowledge about particular breast cancer genes, women with breast cancer can live longer or survive their cancers. They are often confronted, however, with multiple surgeries such as double mastectomies, hysterectomies and reconstruction, as well as treatments such as chemotherapy, radiation therapy and other invasive, long-term medical therapies that can be accompanied by additional disability and emotional suffering. This chapter centers on the knitted sculpture and embroidery of craft artist Christine Carey. Carey stitched painstakingly accurate embroideries of her breast cancer journey onto old-fashioned doilies and her knitted soft sculpture of her eight cupcake breasts. Carey juxtaposed her psychological vulnerability, illustrated by the delicate doilies, with the invasiveness of the surgical knife of her mastectomy, which she depicted through the sharp embroidery needle. Through her artwork, the artist was able to transform her losses into objects that could instill new meaning for women with breast cancer. In the second half of the chapter, Suzanne Isken contextualizes Carey's art by discussing how other artists, including Joseph Bueys and Hannah Wilke, used arts and crafts to document their journeys with physical illness. Suzanne also explores how viewers can be psychologically impacted when seeing these works of art as part of a museum exhibition.

In Chapter 4, *Cutting, Pasting and Piercing: A Memoir*, the writer and artist Corinne Lightweaver shares her painful experience of mastectomy and breast reconstruction. A two-time cancer survivor, Lightweaver's colorful collages and sculpture draw upon both conscious memories and unconscious fragments that surfaced during her treatment. These powerful creative inner mirrors projected onto collages give the viewer insights into Lightweaver's strong emotions, externalizing her inner images and transforming them into powerful art pieces. Derrida might call these renderings strong "autobiographical inscriptions" (Derrida). Many breast cancer survivors will be able to identify with her powerful imagery and the strong accompanying affects that brought them forth.

Chapter 5, entitled *Remembering, Creating and Working Through*, takes its inspiration from Sigmund Freud's essay titled *Remembering, Repeating and Working-Through* (1914). By changing Freud's "Repeating" to "Creating," this chapter demonstrates how long-standing childhood psychological traumas can resurface during cancer treatment, but also how art therapy in the context of cancer treatment can help a patient confront past traumas in productive and healing ways. In this essay, lawyer, artist and writer Loene Trubkin discusses how the supportive and safe transitional space of the *Cancer and Creativity Group* both helped her to deal with the difficulties of her cancer treatments and experiences, while also giving her new tools with which to confront long-standing traumatic memories from her emotionally deprived childhood. For Loene, the process of creating art in an accepting and free-floating group opened up a creative space between the individual and the environment. This new space provided her with a sense of freedom to experiment with color and forms. Similar to the poems and writing she wrote at home, the acrylic paintings she produced in the art group allowed her to transform her dark childhood moods into colorful depictions of the natural environment of the county where she lived as a child. She gained insights that she then was able work though with her personal psychoanalyst in weekly private sessions.

Chapter 6, *Art As Life-Saver*, showcases Zizi Raymond's art installation about the challenges of eating with cancer. The initial idea of focusing on food and weight fluctuation is part of the cancer experience developed out of conversations and early experimental works in the art workshop. The artist, a long-term breast cancer survivor, had lost significant amounts of weight after one of her many complicated surgeries. Through giving voice and vision to her concerns about eating—through a combination of Facebook posts and cellphone photography—Raymond was able to start eating again and, eventually, to gain weight. It also, however, allowed her to come to terms with her body's gradual weakening. Zizi's renewed focus on art made her slow physical decline more psychologically bearable. It ushered in a real transformation in her artistic expression and in her relationship to her body. Zizi Raymond succumbed to breast cancer in 2014 after a 22-year struggle with the disease. In this chapter, Raymond's younger sister, Devon, explains the genesis of this installation and reflects on the impact that it had on her sister's relationship to her illness in the final years of her life, followed by my own associations about the installation process of this art project.

Chapter 7, *Understanding My Wonderland-ing: Sharing my Brain Tumor Experience*, features the writing of photographer, video artist and dance therapist Ashley Myers-Turner. Though Myers-Turner was not a member of the art therapy group, she created in her photographic images the symptoms of her malignant brain tumor before, during and after diagnosis. Her digital collages capture the out-of-body experiences she endured before her diagnosis, which she describes as both scary and confusing, and also funny and embarrassing. During the active period of her illness and after her brain surgery, Ashley took photographic digital self-portraits while looking into the mirror. These self-portraits transformed her threatening experience into a more creative and less upsetting one. Using the imaginary, Ashley was able to make use of the disconcerting, frightening bodily perceptions and symptoms, counteracting her fears of psychic fragmentation and disintegration. They also bridged the gap of her experience of a fragmented, seizured self and the self she encountered in the mirror. Ashley also shared these digital collage self-portraits with her neurologist, family members and close friends. Doing so allowed her caregivers to understand the impact of her cancer symptoms on her psyche and her daily life and to access her suffering in new ways. This, in turn, provided them with ideas about how to help in ways that they were unable to beforehand. The acts of creating and sharing her digital collages not only engendered insight they also allowed her to transform her fragmented self into a more integrated one. As she saw herself through the mirror, Ashley was able to create a new identity for herself and others that fostered reparation and transformation. This chapter uses Ashley's self-portraits as a springboard for exploring the use of the camera and photography as a creative tool and draws on theoretical discussions of Lacan's mirror stage and the imaginary as it relates to Winnicott's transitional object.

Chapter 8, *Cancer Maps and Super Heroes*, focuses on art therapy groups with children and teenagers who are battling cancer or have survived cancer. The chapter begins by addressing the common psychological and psychosocial issues that come up for children who have cancer, as well as those faced by their parents and siblings. Today, pediatric cancers are often curable, but they may include long periods of chemotherapy and multiple surgeries, thus engendering major temporary trauma in children as well as their siblings and parents. In one art therapy group, a group of children created *Cancer Maps* of their cancer journey; in another, they painted and pasted fabric on big canvases portraying themselves as their personal superheroes. Not only were these children encouraged to write a small description about their pictures, but they were also taught how to discuss their art pieces within the group setting. In some groups, the young children were assigned a "paintbrush partner," an older, healthy high school student who helped them execute their ideas. This idea applied art therapist Edith Kramer's theory of the third hand as a supporting one. This chapter illustrates how important it is for children and teenagers with cancer to express their personal cancer journeys pictorially in order to illustrate—and thus recognize—their fears as well as their hopes. It is especially important to understand and analyze the physical and psychological impact on their bodies and on their self-image, which can affect their moods. The power of artistic expression and of understanding these art pieces can help repair the child's injured self after intrusive surgeries or chemotherapies and guide their parents and siblings to a better understanding of their suffering as well as the secondary gains that can come from their journey as cancer warriors.

Chapter 9, *Cancer! Life is going on any Anyway*, addresses the reality that when patients confront cancer treatment, it does not necessarily mean that all their other life issues suddenly disappear. Financial worries, aging or dying parents, unempathetic friends, the health challenges of family members, miscommunications with doctors, work-related problems and survivor's guilt often compound cancer trauma, making it more emotionally complex for the patient to be relaxed enough to focus fully on their cancer journey. This chapter features Mary E. Walter's series of paper cutouts as well as her comic book series, titled *Not 'Cancery Enough': From Track Pants to Yoga Pants*. Walter, a special-effects Hollywood film editor, uses the playful aesthetic forms of the cutout and the comic strip along with narrative humor to relieve some of her fears and anxieties and foster hope for a less traumatic future. Walter writes in this chapter about how the Creativity and Cancer Group, as well as a parallel class in which she learned to draw and write comic books, inspired her to make a comic book about her cancer journey. These comic books address her experience with melanoma skin cancer and her experience of the art therapy group. Perhaps because Mary spent so much time looking at motion picture images, one frame at a time, laid out on a light box in the company of professional storytellers, she got interested in arranging the individual "frames" of the comic book, called panels. In this chapter, Mary struggles with the idea that she might not be sick enough for a cancer support group, as her symptoms were more hidden, unlike her cancer friends' cohort. In dialogue with Walter, I discuss the different defense mechanisms and fears that group members can develop as they are confronted with other members in the group who are in more advanced stages of cancer. Drawing out her picture stories one panel at the time helped this artist keep a healthy distance, to understand her own behaviors and to process her other traumatic experiences with family and doctors. Through these artistic projects, Walter was able to capture her physical and psychological trauma, restore her self-confidence and eventually to refocus on her professional life outside of the cancer community.

Chapter 10, *Art and Death and Mourning*, draws on personal, clinical and psychoanalytic literature about terminal care to discussions on the role of art in transference and countertransference issues as they become manifest in the preterminal and terminal stages of cancer. In the final stages of cancer, both patients and therapists are forced to make tremendous inner changes as multiple mourning processes are activated. By highlighting short case vignettes of adult cancer patients, this chapter demonstrates how art can be used by a patient as a way to work through this intensely painful and, by the end, often ambivalent loss, as well as by the art therapist who mourns for her deceased patient. In the course of the psychoanalytic art-psychotherapy of critically ill or dying cancer patients, an externalization of ego functions becomes necessary, as external relationships keep changing and the patient becomes weaker and is much more self-focused. Creating and exhibiting the art of more terminal cancer patients can be rewarding and informative not only for the artists, the therapist, the oncologists and their families and friends; these images also can communicate important psychological insights about the terminal care of people with cancer for the greater community of viewers.

In Chapter 11, *Art and Cancer in the Public Space*, museum director and curator Suzanne Isken focuses on the dialogue between the artist with cancer and the gallery or museum viewer, who might question what art is and who the insider or outsider is. She discusses other artists who used their art to deal with their cancer and who exhibited it in museum settings, analyzing the empathic reaction of the audience. She suggests that these exhibitions make feelings manifest that most often are hidden to the unaware viewer. To view "cancer art" requires the viewer to confront uncomfortable truths, exposing illness, trauma, death and dying. These are themes that most people would prefer not to confront, as they can destabilize our own sense of security and health. The author discusses how artists with cancer hope to educate the public about their illness as well as the physical and psychological traumas connected to it through their aesthetic manifestations. They hope not only to transform their own experiences with illness but also those of their viewers. Iskin discusses the importance of the presentation and installation of these art works because the way that they are curated helps to foster dialogues between the artist and the viewers.

The Appendix, *Scribble, Squiggle, Doodle, Cut and Paste: creative transformation through creative play at home*, lists creative exercises matched with proposed materials for patients to play creatively at home, as unfortunately not every cancer patient has the chance to attend a Cancer and Creativity group or can participate in Art Therapy in a local Cancer Center.

Bibliography

Bion, W. (1967). Notes on memory and desire. *The Psychoanalytic Forum*, II(3), 271–280.

Bohleber, W. (2011). Exploring core concepts: Sexuality, dreams and the unconscious. *The International Journal of Psycho-Analysis*, 92(2), 285–288.

Copjec, J. (2002). *Imagine there's no woman*. Boston, MA: Beacon Press.

Ehrenzweig, A. (1965 [1999]). *The psycho-analysis of artistic vision and hearing: An introduction to a theory of unconscious perception*. New York: Psychology Press.

Ehrenzweig, A. (1967 [1988]). *The hidden order of art: A study in psychology of artistic perception*. London: Phoenix Press.

Deane, K., Fitch, M., & Carman, M. (2000). An innovative at therapy program for cancer patients. *Canadian Oncology Nursing Journal*, 10, 147–157.

Foucault, M. (1963 [2003]). *The birth of the clinic: An archeology of medical perception*. Translated by A. M. Shedrian Smith. London and New York: Routledge, p. 145, 83.

Foucault, M. (1973 [1994]). *Madness and civilazion*. Translated by A. M. Sheridan Smith. New York: Vintage Books; Random House, Inc.

Geue, K., Goetze, M., Buttstaedt, E., Kleinert, D., Richter, D., & Singer, S. (2010). An overview of arts therapy interventions for cancer patients and the results of the research. *Complementary Therapies in Medicine*, 18(3–4), 160–170.

Lacan, J. (1954). *The ego in Freud's theory and in the technique of psychoanalysis. 1954–55*. The seminars of Jacques Lacan. Book II (1978). Edited by J.-A. Miller, translated by S. Tomaselli. New York: Norton.

Lacan, J. (1966). *Écrits: The first complete edition in English*. Translated by B. Fink. New York: Norton.

Lacan, J. (1973). *The four fundamental concepts for psycho-analysis*. The seminar of Jacque Lacan. Book XI (1981). Edited by J.-A. Miller, translated by Alan Sheridan. New York: Norton.

Lacan, J. (1977). "The mirror stage as formation of the function of the I as revealed in psychoanalytic experience." In *Écrits: A selection*. Translated by Alan Sheridan. New York: W.W. Norton and Company.

Langer, S. (1953). *Feeling and form*. New York: Charles Scribner's Sons

Laub, D., & Podell, D. (1995). Art and trauma. *The International Journal of Psycho-Analysis,* 76(5), 991–1005.

Merleau-Ponty, M. (1964). "Eye and mind." In *The primacy of perception*. Edited by J. M. Edie. Evanston, IL: Northwestern University Press, pp. 159–190.

Merleau-Ponty, M. (1945 [1962]). *Phenomenology of perception*. Translated by C. Smith. London and New York: Routledge.

Nainis, N., Paice, J.A., Ratner, J., Wirth, J.H., Lai, J., & Shott, S. (2006). Relieving symptoms in cancer: Innovative use of art therapy. *Journal of Pain & Symptom Management*, 31(2), 162–169.

Navarro, Z. (2006). In search of a cultural interpretation of power: The contribution of Pierre Bourdieu. *Institute of Development Studies Bulletin*, 37(6), 11–22.

Reineman, J. (2011). Between the imaginary and the real: Photographic portraits of mourning and of melancholia in Argentina. *The International Journal of Psycho-Analysis*, 92(5), 1241–1261.

Reynolds, F., & Prior, S. (2006). The role of art making in identity maintenance: Case studies of people living with cancer. *European Journal of Cancer Care*, 15(4), 333–341.

Rilke, R.M. (1945). *Letters of Rainer Maria Rilke: 1892–1910*. Translated by J. B. Greene and M. D. Herter Norton. New York: W.W. Norton & Co, p. 285.

Schwab, G. (1994). *Subjects without selves: Transitional texts in modern fiction*. Cambridge, MA: Harvard University Press.

Sedofsky, L. (1994). *Being in numbers: Interview with the artist and philosopher Alain Badiou by Lauren Sedofsky*, Art Forum October 1994, p. 82.

Ulrich, C.M. (2013). Who am I? Reflections on self-image among patients with cancer in clinical trials. *Clinical Journal of Oncology Nursing*, 17(6), E68–E70.

Visser, A., & Hoog, M. (2008). Education of creative art therapy to cancer patients: Evaluation and effects. *Journal of Cancer Education*, 23(2), 80–84.

Winnicott, D.W. (1971) *Playing and reality*. New York: Basic Books.

Wacquant, L., & Bourdieu, P. (1992). *An invitation to reflexive sociology*. Chicago, IL: Chicago University Press.

Wood, M.J.M., Molassiotis, A., & Payne, S. (2011). What research evidence is there for the use of art therapy in the management of symptoms in adults with cancer? A systematic review. *Psycho-oncology*, 20(2), 135–145.

Chapter 1

Sigmund Freud's consultation room and the art studio

Potential spaces for creative transformation

Esther Dreifuss-Kattan and Corinne Lightweaver

This chapter compares Sigmund Freud's iconic consultation room—located first in Vienna and then, after the start of the Second World War, in London, where patient and analyst would have been surrounded by many collected artifacts, small sculptures, images, reliefs and carpets—to the art studio-*atelier*, where artist-patients meet in a group with the art-psychotherapist to create art, while exploring their lives with cancer and its treatments. These artist-patients have been faced, suddenly, with new realities and visited with unsettling medical trauma. They meet in the space of the art room for creative exploration and play, ultimately to work through and, eventually, integrate their traumatic experiences. Not unlike Freud's patients on the couch who were asked to free associate verbally with memories of their pasts in order to help them access their unconscious, cancer patients free associate by painting, drawing or making cutout collages in a safe and creative environment. The art-psychotherapist is there to catalyze this free play of the imagination, not unlike Freud, though in a somewhat less tactile and messy fashion.

When we look at furnished, intimate spaces like Freud's consultation room, with its sculptures and couch, and the art studio, with its art supplies, pictures and social interaction, we recognize certain common features, some perhaps paradoxical. These spaces can be isolated but are penetrable as well, open for patients and artist but closed to others. While they may usually be very private, they also open to the public at other times. Moreover, within these two spaces their occupants partake of particular slices of biographical time. While Edward Soja (1989, p. 11) addresses spatiality more in geographical and social terms, he also makes us aware that life stories have their own geography, with their own milieu, with places internal to their narratives and locales where biography takes on a particular dialectic of space, time and social being. The spatialization of personal history results in a human geography. The consultation room and the art space encompass psychosocial life, connecting the enclosure of a particular spatial aesthetic to seeing, hearing, talking and creating.

In his essay "Of Other Spaces," Michel Foucault (1986, p. 29) addresses public spaces opening onto one another, using the metaphor of the "Mirror for Utopia." He claims that the image that you see in the mirror does not really exist, but the mirror itself is a real object that shapes the way we relate to our own image. In Freud's consultation room there is a similar mirror in the reflections of the psychoanalyst, with his ability to show patients their conscious and unconscious state of mind, the sometimes hidden or overlooked forces affecting their life and relationships. In the art studio, conversely, the patient looks into the mirror of his or her own creations, associating and telling a story that reflects on a particular mood and personal psychological mapping, tracing in artistic media the genealogy of their mental states and uncovering an archaeology of causes. Both the consultation room and the art studio are enveloping spaces, rooms of self-representation that reach a unique depth of vision (Soja, 1989, p. 11).

Sigmund Freud's consultation room

The well-known photographs taken by Edmund Engelman in May 1938 of Sigmund Freud's home and office spaces in Berggasse 19 in Vienna, where Freud had worked and lived since 1891, document in detail the iconic consultation room as it stood before Freud's escape from the Nazis. Engleman, M. (1976) Freud used the consulting room for almost 30 years, centering its space on the couch alongside the wall and opposite the window. Freud received the couch from a patient in 1890 (Welter, 2012a); it was covered with oriental rugs and another rug was hung behind the wall to protect it. With the chair behind it, the couch formed the core element of this unprecedented, but now iconic, configuration of psychoanalytic treatment. In "On the Beginning of Treatment" (1913), Freud explains that his earlier treatment of hypnosis was the origin of the patient's horizontal position on a couch, preserving professional discretion by allowing the doctor to hide his facial reactions from the patient. Freud called it "a certain ceremonial of the situation in which the treatment is carried out" (Freud, 1913/1955). Freud set up his new working and living spaces in exile in London 1939 in the exact same way. His daughter Anna Freud, who had her own consultation room in the same house, later turned this location into the Freud Museum, as we know it today in the Hampstead area of London.

Freud modeled his office in Vienna in part after his mentor and teacher, the French psychiatrist Jean-Martin Charcot, a world-renowned neurologist and brilliant educator with whom Freud worked at the Salpêtrière Hospital in Paris when he was 29 years old. Charcot was to have an unparalleled influence on the young Freud, stimulating a lifelong interest in the arts that foreshadowed the career not only of his son Ernst, an architect, but also that of artistic grandson, the famous English painter Lucian Freud. Charcot also published a series of uncanny photographs in the early 1880s at the Salpêtrière Hospital of women with a "social disturbance" later called hysteria. These images were not artistic expressions as such, but rather "scientific experiments" using the newly invented flash to highlight a "new" pathology through a new type of pictorial documentation. Charcot's reliance on the image in his research on hysteria would influence Freud's professional career as much as the now familiar layout of Charcot's consultation room (Baer, 2005).

Charcot collected Chinese and Indian antiquities that he displayed with other artifacts in his expansive living and working spaces in Paris. In a letter dated January 20, 1886, that Freud sent to his fiancée Martha Bernays, he evokes the aesthetic of Charcot's home in a way that now seems telling:

> The other section [of his apartment] has a fireplace..., a table and cases containing Indian and Chinese antiques.... The walls are covered with goblins and pictures, the walls themselves are painted terra cotta... the same wealth of pictures, goblins, carpets and curios—in short a museum.
>
> (Freud, 1885)

Charcot's collection of exotic objects, like the collection of Egyptian and Near Eastern antiquities in the museum in Paris created for Freud a "dreamlike world" (Letters of Sigmund Freud, p. 194). Freud echoes these sentiments in 1922 in a letter to his friend and colleague, the Hungarian psychoanalyst Sandor Ferenczi, where he expresses again this particular emotion prompted by his collecting of small antique sculptures: a "strange secret yearning, perhaps from my ancestral heritage, for the Orient and the Mediterranean and for a life of quite another kind: wishes from late childhood never fulfilled and not adapted to reality" (Gay, 1988, n. 4).

Freud bought his first antiques in 1896, two months after his father's death, when, at age 40 he decorated his first office, shortly before he started his self-analysis (Bergstein, 2003). "I may say once that I am no connoisseur in art, but simply a layman... Nevertheless, works of art do exercise a powerful effect on me" (Freud, 1914, p. 211). In the milieu of turn-of-the-century Vienna, archaeology, a very new field of investigation, had just become an influence on bourgeois taste, recommending its objects of investigation as equally aesthetic ones for home furnishing. By 1938, Freud had collected more than 2,000 ancient objects, half of them from Egypt and the rest mostly from Greece and Rome (Corcoran, 1991). Freud writes to his friend Fliess in January 30, 1899, that: "for relaxation I am reading Burckhart's History of Greek civilization, which is providing me with unexpected parallels. My predilection for the prehistoric in all its human form has remained the same" (Anzieu, 1986, p. 412). In a letter to another friend, the writer Stephan Zweig, he observes that he actually reads more archaeology than psychology (Freud & Zweig, 1970). Freud's office and consultation room formed a virtual museum, dark and crowded, the floors covered with Oriental carpets that were also draped on tabletops and, as mentioned, on his couch. The walls were lined with bookcases, framed photographs, engravings, sculptural reliefs and mounted fragments. Freud's working desk, tabletops, shelves and cabinets were filled with small-scale Greek, Roman and Egyptian figurines (Kurtz, 1986). Freud amassed this collection between 1896 and 1939, most of which were small sculptures from Egypt, Greece, Ancient Rome and China, as well as the Near East.

Most of the Egyptian figurines were shown in frontal view, conforming to ancient Egyptian canons of representation; Freud also lined up these figures on his writing desk facing him. Most of these small, sharp-edged Egyptian sculptures are *shabtis* and *ushabti*, magical objects that were mass-produced by anonymous artisans and made from metal, stone and ceramics. They are votive figures, offerings to the gods for funerary use, intended for magical and religious purposes and placed in ancient Egyptian tombs. Often inscribed with lines from chapter six of the Book of the Dead, a *shabti*, which translates as "answerer," was thought to animate, and specifically to serve, the souls of the deceased, should they be called to the netherworld (http:emol. org/kabbalah/ushabti/). Freud loved these objects as they embodied a continuity with the Egyptian and Greco-Roman mythologies from which he developed some of his psychoanalytic theory. He equated the deciphering of their inscriptions to the interpretation of dreams, using these antiquities as a metaphor for the new science of psychoanalysis as it argued that dreams, fantasies and neuroses preserve atavistic mental or psychic tendencies (*seelische Altertuemer*) (Freud, 1916, p. 371, Kuspit, 1989, pp. 133–151). The psychoanalyst becomes an archaeologist as he excavates multiple deep layers of the patient's psyche to uncover valuable treasures.

Freud also enjoyed the visual and tactile pleasure he received from handling small antique sculptures. He rearranged them often on his desk and at the dining table they sometimes became animated companions. It is well documented that the sculptures were not only used by Freud as decorative artifacts in his working room and consultation space but were also intimately present in his life outside of it. When Freud moved to his summer residence outside Vienna, these objects were packed up by his wife and sent along with him. Perhaps they kept him company, connecting him to his creative inner space and his home office or inspiring his intellectual, psychoanalytic pursuits (Scully, 1997).

Walter Benjamin, the German literary critic, essayist and philosopher, writes that the collector's passion "borders on the chaos of memories" (Benjamin, 1968, p. 60); Benjamin was himself was an avid collector of books and children's toys. Touching the pieces with his hands, Benjamin writes, the collector feels like he touches the world, acquires knowledge, recovers personal experience, and moves another's soul. The touching of and looking at objects or images allows for a particular intimacy and closeness, a more practical remembering, a window through which to view and to understand the past. For Benjamin, handling objects can jumpstart thinking, weaving the chaos of memory into the linear passage of time, and creating a new concept of one's past, intertwined with the threads of the present (Leslie, 1998). Benjamin discusses in his essay how artists and children also love to collect, perhaps with a naïve desire to redeem a past world as if it were like painting a picture or cutting out a figure and preserving it in a portfolio for later viewing. "Relationships to objects and images can be mysterious and speak to a deep desire for the renewal of the old with the new" (Benjamin, 1968, p. 60). Benjamin's observations are as true for Freud as for the artists I work with in my cancer groups.

In addition to their value as touchstones that induce memories, Freud's statuettes also may have possessed magical, totemic powers for him, as their origins suggest. He once apparently deliberately threw and broke a small marble sculpture of Venus in 1905 when his daughter Martha was gravely ill; another time he threw a sculpture in an attempt to repair a friendship that was threatened (Yerushalmi, 1991). Freud, like Benjamin's artist or child, experienced his art collection as a source of exceptional, even miraculous, renewal, *Erquickung* in German, an "invigoration" (Gay, 1988, p. 171).

Like the scholar's study or the art studio, Freud's working space was created and invented by him: it was and is a *Gesamtkunstwerk*, an all-inclusive artistic creation or a synthesis of the arts, an environment to showcase his interest in literature and the arts. He writes in his introduction to the essay "The Moses of Michelangelo" that "works of art do exercise a powerful effect on me, especially those of literature and sculpture, less often of painting" (Freud, 1914, p. 211). To this end, Mary Bergstein wonders if Freud wrote most about sculpture because of the contrast between its hard, monumental durability and the "softer" concepts, such as dreams and memories, of his day-to-day work treating his patients (Bergstein, 2003, p. 3).

Freud's first visit to Rome in 1897, together with his brother Alexander, provides an example of this "powerful effect," and it was accompanied by major angst perhaps rooted in his upbringing. He wrote to his wife that there were heavy storms in Rome, so terrible and overwhelming that they "could have been created by Michelangelo" himself (Bergstein, 2010, p. 65). It was on this trip that Freud first visited the actual sculpture of Moses by Michelangelo in the church of San Pietro in Vincoli which would inspire the essay by the same name; the statue sits like an idol (or figurine) of sorts on Paul Julius's tomb. (Mahagoni, 2006) Freud wrote to his friend and collaborator Fliess on December 3, 1897 that "my longing for Rome...is deeply neurotic," though he could reminisce, four years later that his first visit had been "overwhelming for me … a high point of my life" (Masson, 1985). When, also in 1901, Freud saw the Acropolis for the first time he wrote that he was moved to feelings of "derealization extraordinary, almost hallucinatory" (Yerushalmi, 1991, p. 76). Both of these experiences of spectatorship might have brought forth

Freud's inner, somewhat repressed tensions with his late father, whose Jewish name was Jacob Moses and who, as an orthodox Jew, might not have approved of Freud's obsession with an image of Moses or with pagan religious iconography. Freud's particular interests in collecting Egyptian and Greek sculpture set the stage for the expansion of the lives of his descendants to a more general, transcultural identification with more universal archetypes than those of psychoanalytic technique. With the many artifacts, sculptures, ancient reliefs and prints he collected, Freud might also have wanted to signal to himself, and to his family, patients and friends a more expanded, enlightened cultural background. Already in 1865, the nine-year-old Freud entered the Leopoldstaedler Communal Gymnasium in Vienna, where he studied Greek and Latin, learning to embrace a new culture and the idols forbidden to him by his religious upbringing (Ostow, 1989, p. 483).

Sigismund, as Sigmund Freud was called as a boy, received his first Bible when he was seven years old and studied it with his father, handling it so often that it required a new leather binding when his father Jacob presented it again to him again for his 37th birthday (Ostow, 1989). Freud writes in his Autobiography: "My deep engrossment in the Bible story (almost as soon as I learned the art of reading) had, as I recognized much later, an enduring effect upon the direction of my interest" (Freud, 1925, p. 8). This sophisticated Bible was a synthesis of original Hebrew text with a German translation and erudite Talmudic commentary, an apparatus that commented on thematic references to surrounding cultures and a generous amount of woodcut engraving of Egyptian, Greco-Roman, early Christian and 18th- and 19th-century Romantic images. The illustrations also included lithographs of Middle Eastern landscapes, animals and botanicals, all executed in a nostalgic, Orientalist tradition influenced by 19th-century taste.

Freud's early exposure to this book, the Philippson Bibel, *Die Heilige Schrift Der Israeliten* or "The Holy Scripture of the Israelites," most likely also informed the manner in which Freud collected and exhibited his sculptures in his office. The Philippson Bibel is a densely, multiculturally illustrated Jewish Bible (also known as the Old Testament or The Five Books of Moses) that he explored together with his father in his early childhood and which left him with memories of warmth and excitement. The Philippson Biebel's translator, Dr. Ludwig Philippson, was a university-educated scholar, writer and rabbi, who lived in Magdeburg Germany and completed a reformed family Bible together with his brother Phoebus in 1854.

Researchers believe that Freud's collection of Egyptian and other ancient sculpture must have tapped into the pictorial psychic archive of his childhood, an archive formed when Freud stored these early illustrations of the Philippson Bibel in his optical unconscious. Collecting, exhibiting, sharing and handling these statuettes might have aroused similar affective, tactile excitement and satisfaction, integrating his past with the present, as well as tapping into a collective unconscious that transcends personal religion and contemporary culture (Whitebrook, 2010). Freud's collection of antiquities, placed in his consultation room and office spaces, might have been his way to bind together fragments of his own past, connecting a perhaps childishly naïve ambition, the science of psychoanalysis, to the childhood imagery in the Philippson Bibel stored in his psyche, and "renovated" by the new science of archeology.

Through Freud's technique of free associations and transference in the otherworldly cave-like consultation room, he allowed himself and his patients access to inner transitional experiences, recovering the fragments of the past behind their affective perceptions. The room's ambience suspended the opposition of past to present, fostering the primitive merger that allowed patients to recover psychic cohesion, all nonetheless within the well-defined framework of a session. That is, Freud provided for the patients who lay across his Persian carpets the intermediate space of a room-*cum*-museum, and the curios therein encouraged the free-floating attention that could yield up the *trouvailles* of unconscious memory and creative thought. The consultation room, then, achieves a "symbiotic aesthetic" with the analytic session; the analytic room, Kurtz explains, can become a transformational object (Bollas, 1979), a transformation that inspires reverence, a "sacred space" not unlike the art studio (Kurtz, 1986, p. 48).

The art studio and art therapy room: a space for creative transformation

Freud seemed to pass on his preoccupation with art to his youngest son, Ernst (1892–1970), who became a successful domestic architect in the Weimar Republic, and later in London after 1933. Ernst was the first of Freud's children born in the Berggasse 19 apartment in Vienna and used to pass the time in his father's office and consultation room, witnessing the buildup of Freud's collection first-hand and the images of ancient cities on its walls. His father's obsession with archaeology most likely influenced Ernst's choice of profession.

In the German architectural monthly called *"The Pyramide"* published in 1928, we see a photo of a domestic interior created by Ernst Freud, accompanied by an article called: *"Zu Hause"* [At Home]. It asserts that the *zu hause*, the being at home, has to keep at bay the questionable, wicked, threatening and alien outside world. He writes:

> The 'Zu Hause' [At Home] begins with early childhood. ...Here within the security, the child begins to grasp thankfully and with fresh senses the environment. How constructive childhood impressions are! The pattern of wallpaper, the form of a table is transformed into unheard of experiences. Such memories remain at work in the realm of the unconscious, and even with thirty years of age we experience their undiminished influence each time we are about to make a choice.
>
> (Welter, 2012a, p. 8, 90)

The art therapy space and art studio is an agent for transformation for artists with cancer and cancer survivors. Not unlike Freud's consultation room, or the *Zu Hause* "at Home" of Ernst Freud's architecture, it can become a comfortable place for free association, fostering creative thinking, opening up imagination and finding new forms and solutions to new real-life problems. Freud's couch is replaced in the art room by a large art table that brings the group together and also seats the art-psychotherapist. The art studio also includes art supplies, such as different kinds and colors of paper, canvas and fabric, providing stimuli for free association and access to the unconscious. The art studio, like the consultation room, opens the possibility of creation and transition, of sharing the past in the present and looking toward the future.

The art studio, or *atelier*, is thus a safe space with its own personal aesthetic (Salazar, 2014). As an actively contributing space, it helps cancer patients and survivors to realize their creative potential while contemplating illness and health, cancer and its treatments, fears of reoccurrence and life and death. "Drawing out" and "leading forth," terms coined by Ault and Beck, fit here well. (Ault & Beck, retrieved: www.manifest.org/docs/05.pdf) "Drawing out" means encouraging our patient-artists to realize their creative potential and to get in touch with their own artistry, their emotional, social and cultural context and their fears and hopes. "Leading forth" describes the quiet guidance the art-psychotherapist extends to patient-artists as they slowly work through their belated trauma of cancer and its treatments in conference with other group members. Leading forth aims to integrate these experiences and traumata; only then can the patient-artist rejoin emotionally with their social world, first within the group and later with family, friends and the world at large. Art making opens up a dialogue with the outside world and in the process facilitates a more stable, integrated sense of self and a new sense of belonging.

O'Doherty writes that "The artist studio stands for the art, … the artist for the process, the product for the artist, the artist for the studio" (O'Doherty, 2008, p. 6). The circular structure O'Doherty outlines here is useful for us: it is the art therapy space that contains and protects the artist-patient, fostering the creative process by which they form the content of their life with illness. This formed content, the art piece, then provokes discussion and insight that can be shared and contemplated with other patient-artists in the group, refreshing and renewing the protective powers of the space. Holistically, this circular process encourages reflection and the sharing of creative ideas and strong feelings, inspiring other artists to go beyond their expressive comfort zones. Amidst this process, the art therapist tries to support the notion of individuality, appreciating everybody's uniqueness both as artists and as cancer patients, while also seeding the bonds of a strong cohort and tracking its group dynamics. Both the art studio and the psychoanalyst consultation room foster creative and intellectual inquiry, as well as psychological reflection within a spatial context and with specific rituals. Both the studio and consultation room can change into "imagination chambers" that "make visible what has been seen but has not yet been looked at" (O'Doherty, 2008, p. 6). Fostering connection and belonging as well as encouraging ideas and experimentation with different art material and concepts, this new social, therapeutic group of patient-artists with different cancers engenders collaborative empowerment and encouragement (Sullivan, 2009).

Much like the creative incubator of the artist collective, the art therapy space encourages dialogue, facilitates trust and finds common themes— here of the patient-artist experience with many different types of cancer— all while inculcating sensitivity to aesthetic values (Salazar, 2014). This room for exploration and creative play allows a new sense of identity to surface, that of an artist and not solely that of a person with cancer. The images and sculpture created might relate inside, the psyche, to outside, the social environment of illness and health. The art room, the agent of protection and creation, with its therapist facilitator can become a safe container for the contextualization of free associations and for creative exploration, a springboard to access one's pictorial memory as well as more hidden unconscious fantasies. This atelier can be made into a protective environment for self-contained absorption, a form of artistic reverie, a holding environment for new exciting ideas as well as overwhelming feelings and trauma.

Because the art therapy space is removed somewhat from the noise and digital intrusions of outside reality, it can turn into the site of coherent personal dialogues between fellow patient-artists that interweave aesthetic ideas with new sensibilities (Sullivan, 2009). It becomes the locus of artistic experimentation, a retreat for contemplative thought and ideas: a spontaneous laboratory for creative inventions. It is like a shared *Spielraum*, or "play-space," where one can touch, pull apart, build or construct with material and forms, like a child in her or his playroom (Loewenberg, 2005). The studio, all in all, is a space of potential, the intermediate area of experiencing what is between fantasy and reality, inside and outside, inducing play, imagination and transformation while fostering symbolization (Winnicott, 1971).

Art making in a creative studio, like free association in a psychoanalytic consultation room, can facilitate the binding together of fragments of memories of the recent or distant past, within a spiritual, physical, artistic and psychological framework. Specifically, the patient-artist can levy his or her good childhood memories against more traumatic ones, using imagination and—unlike the purely psychoanalytic patient—artistic rendering to access traces that have been stored. Occupying this transitional space helps the patient-artist with cancer recover a psychic cohesion that was broken by their potentially life-threatening illness. The freedom that comes with this expanded inner and outer space can be a source of great pleasure, a different kind of creative fulfillment, because, as in the "symbiotic aesthetic" of Freud's consultation room, it is operating between knowledge and unconscious experimentation (Pilgrum, 2007). And, as in the case of Benjamin's collector, touching and working with the various materials and textures of paint, fabric, different kinds of papers, clay or wood can reactivate tactile and physical experiences of the distant past, blurring the divide between present and past, and between self and other. Concentrated engagement with art materials in a safe, inspiring environment expands personal control and authorship over one's own life, an experience that is hard to come by when undergoing cancer treatments.

The studio also plays on the opposition of public and private. Its deliberate barring of information from the outside world can estrange patient-artists from routine perceptions of themselves. They may see themselves, instead, in an uncanny "otherness" that allows them to unpack formerly hidden anger, grief, mourning and "un-thought knowledge" to which their relation has changed (Bollas, 1989, p. 101). The severe physical and psychological limitations that patients face often results in brutal isolation, which can aggravate the fear of death. These fears can take the form of not having enough time; as patients in the studio share this unique and secluded sense of timelessness. These fears can be overcome as the studio is holding them in a sense of timelessness, as if time were standing still. In the place of social isolation, they may feel a comforting fusion. The creative group process, therefore, can initiate personal transformation, through escape from—as well as an encounter with—the time of lived experiences, thus addressing and working through loss, mourning and reparation. At other times the art room or studio can be turned into a public space as the venue for a pop-up art exhibition, allowing the patient-artists an encounter with the other, through family, friends, doctors, nurses or the general public, as well as with their own interiority (Cole & Pardo, 2005).

The writer, artist and cancer patient Corinne Lightweaver, who participated for several years in the Cancer and Creativity group in Santa Monica, shares below her personal experience in the art studio, where we met weekly for art making and creative play:

The hall of mirrors: art making in community

Corinne Lightweaver

Although I was a painter by avocation before my diagnosis with breast cancer in 2007 and lymphoma in 2003, this previous work focused on emotive, wildly colorful depictions of wildlife. From February 2008 to April 2012, I explored my inner world in new ways in the Cancer and Creativity group, and in the process I discovered the medium of collage. This novel method—cutting, pasting and piecing—fit my efforts to piece my body and life back together again.

The process of coming to terms with cancer and its after-effects is long, but it does show sharp transitions. In pulling together the works for an exhibit I was struck by the difference in the descriptions I wrote for the pieces while undergoing the surgical processes in 2008 and 2009, in which the anguish felt so immediate as described in the first person narrative, compared to the descriptions I wrote the following year, which were written in the third person. For the 2010 works, "I" was replaced by "the woman," perhaps symbolizing my movement away from the immediacy of pain, as well as the wish to distance myself from my cancer experience.

Yet when I think about my experience over a three-year period in an art therapy group for cancer patients, the complexity is hard to unravel. It was a period of intense confusion and pain, but also deep discovery. I am not one of those people who say cancer is the best thing that ever happened to me. But I am one who looks to uncover meaning in what one is forced to bear.

Writing about this art therapy experience is difficult. Writing about my cancer experience in a support group for cancer patients was even harder: impossible, actually. I am a writer and make my living working with words. Writing about having cancer was too cerebral and kept me either stilted or just skating the surface of my emotions. Dipping into those same emotions through art, however, opened a different pathway through which I could plumb my unconscious and discover what lay in the depths.

For two hours each week, in a large room bathed in natural light, we members of the art therapy group undertook a shared journey. Some people came and went as inclination or health allowed. Some didn't find what they needed. Some passed away and I still mourn them. The amazing thing for many of us was that the group was free. At a time when we felt overwhelmed financially and emotionally, when we felt cast out of the mainstream of life and less valuable, there was a place just for us, a place where we belonged.

The art room, for me at least, revealed us all like a hall of mirrors. First, there was the mirror of reality: everyone in the room had cancer. Including me. Yes, this was really happening. That was the cold reality of it. But here was the mirror of experience, also. It was not happening to me in isolation. Others were on parallel or intersecting journeys with me. The cancer was happening to me, and that happened on an individual level. But the mirror of experience showed me I was not alone.

Adjacent to the mirror that showed me reality was the mirror that helped me escape reality. They coexisted. In the real world, people who knew I had cancer might always look at me through that lens. Just as I had been afraid or didn't know how to respond to people with cancer before, now I was on the other side of the divide looking at the people I had been. Cancer was a defining marker now that would always separate me from others. But in the art therapy room, there existed a mirror that could help me escape reality. Because when I shared the same identity marker as everyone else in the room, that identity could fall away, in a sense. It was important, but it was less threatening. The "cancer patient" mask that was superimposed on my group mates and me could fall away, allowing us to be individuals with unique experiences and responses.

As one would expect, the art I made itself was also a mirror, but one that reflected much deeper than what lay on the surface. The art I created allowed me to see myself as I truly was in that moment of creating. When I gave myself over to creating, the multilayers and ambiguity fell away—or were exposed in their own right. The independent movement of the hands, the knobby texture of upholstery cloth, the smacking sound of the paint being pulled off the canvas by the brush, the acrid smell of glue and the will to create something as yet unknown from fabric, wood or paper—they all flowed together. For me it was as powerful as when I cooked without a recipe, without an idea of an end product.

But then there was another mirror, or several more. The mirror of the art therapist and her response to my art work; the mirror of my group mates; the mirror of my family and friends when they saw the art work; the response of my doctors when I brought it to them and the response of the public, both those with cancer and those without, when I displayed it at art shows. Having cancer can narrow one's focus. It can narrow one's social interactions. And it can narrow how people respond to you. Creating art established a new pathway for communication: both incoming and outgoing. And interpretation of that artwork by others or myself opened my world again.

Esther Dreifuss-Kattan

Donald W. Winnicott (1971, 1987) explains that cultural objects such as art can negotiate the boundaries between self and the outside world, insofar as they are created in what he called a transitional space. This transitional space, which is originally the first space created between infant and the mother or caregiver. As the infant designates a special toy, blanket or teddy bear and negotiates the mother's temporary absence, Corinne's art and all cultural expressions become transformational objects that can help to contain and bind emotions that would otherwise be too overwhelming.

Medical and psychological trauma can fracture the self and might result in a temporal inability to symbolize. Creating art within a transitional space can bring about a process of transformation of both subjective as well as cultural boundaries, negotiating conscious and unconscious knowledge (Schwab, 2010). Like the culture of Freud's consultation room, the art studio's transitional space is also an analytic one that facilitates recollection, association and the expression of emotions.

References

Anzieu, D. (1986). *Freud's Self-Analysis* (P. Graham, Trans.). Madison, CT: International University Press.

Ault, J., and Beck, M. Drawing Out and Leading Forth. *Manifesto 5*. Retrieved from www.manifest.org/docs/05pdf

Baer, U. (2005). *Spectral Evidence: The Photography of Trauma*. Cambridge, MA: The MIT Press.

Benjamin, W. (1968). Unpacking My Library. In H. Arendt (Ed.), *Illuminations: Essays and Reflections* (pp. 59–68). New York: Schocken Books.

Bergstein, M. (2003). The Dying Slave at Bergstrasse 19. *American Imago, 60*(1), 9–20.

Bollas, C. (1979). The Transformational Object. *International Journal of Psycho-Analysis, 60*, 97–107.

Bollas, C. (1989). *The Shadow of the Object: Psychoanalysis of the Unthought Known*. New York: Columbia University Press, p. 101.

Cole, M., and Pardo, M. (2005). Origins of the Studio. In M. Pardo and M. Cole (Eds.), *Inventions of the Studio: Renaissance to Romanticism*. Chapel Hill: The University of North Carolina Press.

Corcoran, L. H. (1991). Exploring the Archaeological Metaphor: The Egypt of Freud's Imagination. *Annual of Psychoanalysis, 19*, 19–32.

Egyptian Shabtis: An Answer to a Prayer (2016). Retrieved from http:emol.org/kabbalah/ushabti/

Eissler, K. (1976). *Talent and Genius*. New York: Quadrangle Books.

Engleman, E. (1976). *Bergstrasse 19: Sigmund Freud's Home Offices, Viennna 1938: The Photographs of Edmund Engleman*. New York: Basic Books.

Foucault, M. (1986). Of Other Spaces (J. Miskowiec, Trans.). *Diacritics, 16*(1), 22–27.

Freud, S. (1908). Creative Writers and Day-Dreaming. In A. Richards (Ed.), *The Standard Edition of the Complete Psychological Works of Sigmund Freud: Jensen's* Gradiva *and Other Works* (Vol. 9). (J. Strachey, Trans.) (pp. 141–154). London: The Hogarth Press and the Institute of Psychoanalysis.

Freud, S. (1914). The Moses of Michelangelo. In *The Standard Edition of the Complete Psychological Works of Sigmund Freud: Jensen's* Gradiva *and Other Works* (Vol. 9). (J. Strachey, Trans.) (pp. 211–240). London: The Hogarth Press and the Institute of Psychoanalysis.

Freud, S. (1916–1917). Introductory Lectures on Psychoanalysis. In *The Standard Edition of the Complete Psychological Works of Sigmund Freud: Introductory Lectures on Psychoanalysis* (Vols. 15–16). (J. Strachey, Trans.) (pp. 211–236). London: The Hogarth Press and the Institute of Psychoanalysis.

Freud, S. (1957). *Letters of Sigmund Freud* (E. Freud, Ed.). New York: Basic Books, Inc.

Freud, S. (1985). *The Complete Letters of Sigmund Freud to Wilhelm Fliess, 1897–1904* (J. Masson, Ed.). Cambridge, MA: Harvard University Press.

Freud, S., and Zweig, A. (1970). *The Letters of Sigmund Freud and Arnold Zweig.* New York: Harcourt Press.

Gay, P. (1988). *Freud: A Life of Our Time.* New York: W.W. Norton & Company.

Kurtz, S. (1986). The Analyst's Space. *The Psychoanalytic Review, 73*(1), 41–55.

Kuspit, D. (1989). A Mighty Metaphor: The Analogy of Archeology and Psychoanalysis. In L. Gamwell and R. Wells (Eds.), *Sigmund Freud and Art* (pp. 133–151). London: Freud Museum.

Leslie, E. (1998). Walter Benjamin: Traces of Craft. *Journal of Design History, 11*(1), 5–13.

Loewenberg, P. (2005). The Bauhaus as a Creative Playspace: Weimar, Dessau, Berlin, 1919–1933. *Annual of Psychoanalysis, 23,* 209–226.

Mahony, P. J. (2006). The Moses of Michelangelo: A Matter of Solutions. *Canadian Journal of Psychoanalysis, 14,* 11–43.

O'Doherty, B. (2008). *Studio and Cube: On the Relationship between Where Art Is Made and Where Art Is Displayed.* New York: Princeton University Architectural Press.

Ostow, M. (1989). Sigmund and Jacob Freud and the Philippson Bible. *International Review of Psycho-Analysis, 16,* 483–492.

Pigrum, D. (2007). The "Ontology" of the Artist's Studio as Workspace: Researching the Artist's Studio and Art/Design Classroom. *Research in Post-Compulsory Education, 12*(3), 291–307.

Salazar, S. M. (2014). Educating Artists: Theory and Practice in College Studio Art. *Art Education, 67*(5), 32–39.

Scully, S. (1997). Review: Freud's Antiquities: A View from the Couch. *Arion: A Journal of the Humanities and the Classics, 5*(2), 222–233.

Schwab, G. (2010). *Haunting Legacies: Violent Histories and Transgenerational Trauma.* New York: Columbia University Press.

Soja, E. (1989). *Postmodern Geographies: The Reassertion of Space in Critical Social Theory.* London: Verso.

Sullivan, G. (2009). *Art Practice as Research: Inquiry in the Visual Arts* (2nd ed.). London: SAGE Publishing.

Welter, V. M. (2012a). *Ernst L. Freud, Architect: The Case of the Modern Bourgeois Home.* Oxford: Berghahn Books.

Welter, V. M. (2012b, May 6). A House of Franz Alexander's Own. *Berfrois.* Retrieved from www.berfrois.com/2012/03/ernst-freuds-modern-architecture/

Winnicott, D. W. (1971). *Playing and Reality.* New York: Basic Book, Inc.

Winnicott, D. W. (1965). *The Maturational Process and the Facilitating Environment.* New York: International University Press.

Whitebrook, J. (2010). Jacob's Ambivalent Legacy. *American Imago, 67*(2), 139–155.

Yerushalmi, Y. (1991). *Freud's Moses: Judaism Terminable and Interminable.* New Haven, CT: Yale University Press.

Chapter 2

Art as transformational object

Finding form and an aesthetic moment in the transitional space

Esther Dreifuss-Kattan

Artist: Zizi Raymond

I am a slave to my body now. All I ever do now is take care of my body, that's how I spend my time. I am feeding it. Or resting it. Or taking it to the doctor. Which is kind of a nightmare for me because I used to ignore my body.

Zizi Raymond (2009)

So writes Zizi Raymond, a well-known LA artist who battled breast cancer for 20 years. Adam Phillips describes it similarly: "[Illness] narrows our minds, it over-organizes our attention, it prescribes its own limits." – Adam Phillips, "Conversion Hysteria."

I got to know Zizi in 2008 when she came to join the "Cancer and Creativity" group in Santa Monica at the Premiere Oncology Foundation. She later joined the "Healing Arts" group at the University of California, Los Angeles. Her recovery from brain surgery in March 2008 gave Zizi the opportunity to start all over again with her art. Her rehabilitation served as a framework to refocus her art in a new and exciting way. While her previous drawings and sculpture were more figurative, she had always admired more abstract work and found a way to include abstraction as she moved through this new phase of her illness.

In this chapter, I will interpret pieces by Zizi and by other patients, as they relate to the understanding of Winnicott's concepts of transitional phenomena.

The first time I came across Winnicott's book, *Playing and Reality*, was in the summer of 1974, after I had started to work as the first art therapy intern and then the first art therapist at the Chestnut Lodge psychiatric hospital in Rockville, Maryland. Chestnut Lodge had long operated on psychoanalytic principles; established in 1910, it was run for 75 years by the Bullard family, of whom many were psychiatrists. Frieda Fromm-Reichmann, and later Harold Searls, Otto Will, Harry Stack Sullivan, John Kafka, Thomas

McGlashan, Ping Pao and many others treated patients, taught and supervised at Chestnut Lodge, where they tried to understand the individual behind the symptoms they encountered in their psychotic and depressed patients. The famous autobiographical novel, *I Never Promised You a Rose Garden* (1964), written by Joanne Greenberg, a former patient, under the pen name Hanna Green, describes psychoanalytic treatment with Dr. Frieda Fromm-Reichmann. The novel mentions a typical Chestnut Lodge treatment used before tranquilizing medication was developed to calm aggressive patients: Greenberg, who was diagnosed with schizophrenia but today would be called a depressed patient with somatizations, was wrapped very tightly into sheets that were freezing cold, but warmed very fast by her body heat once she relaxed, producing a calming effect. Even when I was at Chestnut Lodge in the 1970s, I witnessed this procedure.

By the time I came from Zurich, Switzerland, Chestnut Lodge had a fully developed version of what we would today call an integrative psychiatry program. Each patient was assigned his or her own psychoanalyst who came to visit in their room. When patients felt better, they could keep appointments at the doctor's office on campus, undergoing four consultations a week of 50 minutes each. Each patient was also assigned a different psychiatrist administrator, who distributed the limited medication available at the time and regulated the patient's privileges in the hospital. This psychiatrist administrator was to decide if a patient could take walks on campus by himself or herself, go into town (with or without a chaperone) or what additional integrative therapy was most helpful for them in a given time. All patients on a given floor had to attend daily group therapy, and some attended dance therapy, music therapy, art therapy, recreational and occupational therapy, or worked in the communal garden and used the gym.

My time at Chestnut Lodge was my first period of travel in the United States; as a good Swiss, I had just terminated my first Jungian analysis, with some Jungian theoretical training behind me, and a year's worth of working in the art studio of the C.G. Jung private psychiatric hospital in Zurich. I immediately realized that I was not prepared for this sophisticated Freudian institution. I was asked to present a new patient after just a few weeks, illustrated by her drawings. She had been diagnosed as a schizophrenic. In front of 40 psychiatrists and psychoanalysts, mostly men, I presented the patient through her art that she had created with me. I addressed the archetypical symbols, the collective unconscious, and while I heard that I should expurgate C.G. Jung's ideas and banish them back to Zurich, I was also commended for my efforts. My audience was duly impressed by how much they learned from these pictures about this particular patient, who had refused to talk to her psychoanalyst, but whose art communicated her internal world very well to me.

I fled to the comprehensive library on the Chestnut Lodge campus, whose compassionate and assiduous librarian guided me through volumes of missing theoretical background, clinical studies and research into Freud and art. At the same time, two of the Chestnut Lodge psychoanalysts, Dr. Goldberg and Dr. Heyt, volunteered to be my weekly supervisors. In our tutorials, I received my most important insights into transference and countertransference, and I prepared to work psychoanalytically with psychotic patients.

Somewhere between the library and my consultations with the staff, I was introduced to Winnicott's then-recent book *Playing and Reality*, which advanced Winnicott's creative theories on the transitional object, transitional phenomena and the idea of the potential space. Marion Milner, an English psychoanalyst and a prominent member of the Independent Psychoanalytic Group in London, together with Winnicott, her supervisor, provide a useful visual symbol for the concept of the potential space.[1] Milner interprets a drawing she did in 1930 that shows the overlapping of two jugs, taking her design as an overlapping of shapes that can be seen as two or one in a given moment (Milner, 1970–1972, 2013). This overlapping space was the exact space I also understood as a theoretical concept: the potential space that contains the art therapy encounter—which is the overlapping communicative efforts of patient and art therapist—crystallizes in the painting as a transitional object. This designated creative space between the patient-artist, the artwork and the psychotherapist was also the space and time when the therapeutic alliance with the patient within the psychoanalytic setting can be built and nurtured. Within this potential space, the patient together with the art therapist can play with symbolization, aesthetic forms and pictorial perception to bring forth fantasies and memories. Milner believed that playing was the only real reality, a belief she ascribed to Winnicott: when people could be creative and play, anything could happen. Milner describes the magic and intimacy that can come from play and reliable relationships. Adam Phillips describes these affordances of play as life-enhancing possibilities over chaos that make life worth living again (Phillips, 2017b).

While simultaneously tracking different affects and behaviors on their journey back to the past within the present, artist-patients can use more than words in expressing the future they experience in transference (Figure 2.1).

One of the early times Zizi took part in one of my groups, I asked the participants to choose boxes of different sizes to create a place for themselves. Zizi decided she wanted to do this project at home and came back the following week with a seven-by-four-and-a-half-inch small box with a lock and a glass front window. She stood it up like a book so we could view black and white slides showing us sick and dismembered body parts through the glass, some bodies with heads and some without. After lifting out the first set of slides, we found two more sheets with six slides, all in black and white and hung like sheets in an armoire. These tiny image collages fitted into the old-fashioned slides with the same content of cut up body parts, which were taken by the patient from an old medical book she had found in a thrift shop.

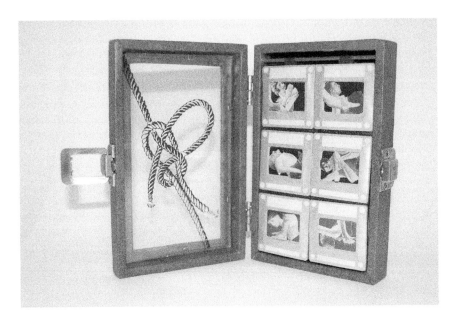

Figure 2.1 Zizi Raymond, "Untitled," 2010, Wood Box with Glass Window and Slides.

Zizi's piece was very creative, delicate and thought-through, and it mimicked a very small doctor's glass vitrine, standing upright with a simple silver or silver-plated lock. It needed few explanations in the group; as she stated above, Zizi was forced by her metastatic cancer to obsess over her body and it took over too much of her time. She might also, however, have communicated a hidden wish to lock this box forever away with its body parts and start all over again, and despite its meticulousness and wry humor about her state, to focus less on cancer and more on art making.

Zizi's vitrine also seemed to have the feeling of a transitional object, poised between this life and the one to come, or between holding on to her artistic control and yielding to her looming fear of loss and mourning. This sculpture was born into a transitional space between the creative, sheltering art therapy group and its therapist/mother and the insecure somatic world outside. It is a very personal sculpture by a talented, introspective artist who could repeatedly identify with her artistic self, transforming illness into a creative act. The work documents the way that despite the multiple physical losses she endured, her choice of art making together with close relationships to her cancer patient friends and her family empowered her to resist depression in the face of her chronic illness.

About eight months before her death, Zizi handed me this sculpture and told me that I should have it, since I had always liked it and, in the first exhibition, we curated together of her and other artists-patients' art-work. This wonderful but uncanny sculpture is a guidepost for me on how art making can be life-affirming and transformational when confronting loss and mourning. It stands on my piano, and it reminds me to exercise my own creativity too.

Winnicott describes how the womb of the mother provides the first environment for the embryo. Once the infant is between a few weeks to 12 months old, the womb is followed by the protective, enveloping environment provided by the mother and/or father. As the parents try to wean the baby from this holding environment, the baby internalizes his or her parents and develops their own personal space, what Winnicott called the "potential space." The potential space becomes an intersubjective, containing space of creative play (Winnicott, 1971). It facilitates the child's early transitions from subjectivity to objectivity—from being merged with the mother to also being separate. These transitional phenomena provide a link between the inner and the outer world, giving the child the ability to be alone in "her space" in a sort of new "state of being," a safe space for symbolizations and play, with a protector, the child having now internalized the containing parent. It is there where the baby creates his or her first not-me possession—a blanket, doll, teddy bear, a transitional object. He or she creates something that offers softness and provides comfort to negotiate separation from the caring adult. Winnicott suggests that later in life the safe, transitional object between self and other turns into artistic and cultural experiences (Ogden, 1985). An art object, be it a painting, a musical composition or some other type, overcomes the frontier between self and other. Hearing a musical composition affects the boundaries of our subjectivity, as well as mediating the cultural boundaries that may isolate us from others (Schwab, 2012).

Winnicott could write, therefore, that "psychotherapy takes place in the overlap of two areas of playing, that of the patient and that of the therapist" (Winnicott, 1971, p. 38). Winnicott was a pediatrician first before becoming a psychoanalyst. He observed mothers with their infants and toddlers, and later took care of displaced children who were sent to the countryside from London during air raids in the Second World War, during which he wrote conclusions about this care-giving dyad, as well as tracking the development of the child. Initially only performing psychoanalysis on children, Winnicott also invented the famous Squiggle technique, making him perhaps the first psychoanalytic art therapist.

Some squiggle drawings were found in Winnicott's notebooks dating from the Second World War, and other squiggles came to light in notebooks dating 20 years later, illustrating his therapeutic work in his consultation room with children (Farley, 2013, p. 418). The projective technique of the Squiggle, which Phillips calls Winnicott's "most famous technical invention" inspired my scribble and doodle technique at Chestnut Lodge in 1974 (Phillips, 1998, p. 15).

In the Squiggle technique, the child or adult would draw a spontaneous squiggle and Dr. Winnicott would add a simple mark to it. Winnicott would then draw his own squiggle and the little patient would add his or her mark to it as well. Both child patient and his or her doctor thus share, here, the creative space of fantasy and free associations, inspiring both play and reverie while gaining insights into each other through co-associating. Generally, the Squiggle technique contributes to patient-therapist mutuality as well to separateness, and, in the process, always illuminates their unconsciousness. This technique was inspired by the mutuality within difference of Freud's dream interpretation, where Freud, after his patients would free associate to dream images, would respond with his own associations, highlighting his patient's early personal history, their symptoms, as well as their day residues surfacing from their dream. Like Winnicott, Freud wanted to get to his patients' memories and associations, both from the recent and far-gone past, in an attempt "to overcome the resistance brought about by repression" (Phillips, 2006, p. 392).

The space and time of free association between art-psychotherapist and patient permits the unfolding of creative forms, memories, feeling and thoughts. The power of the transitional space can then be harnessed: the psychoanalytic art therapy session can turn into a place for a dialectic structure of transference and countertransference while expressive forms and colors spontaneously surface from looking at the art. Wildloecher calls this transitional space "a space in which illusion and creative omnipotence can be experienced as internal reality" (Wildloecher, [2006] 2013, p. 248).

This balance of transference and countertransference, and the unconscious expressive potential of seemingly unrelated aesthetic forms, is well illustrated in Yvonne's picture. Yvonne is a 68-year-old retired professor, mother and grandmother; thin, delicately beautiful and always well dressed, she is also a cancer patient and survivor. In 2017, I asked Yvonne and rest of the Healing Arts group members to create a painting illustrating their personal reaction to a destructive hurricane and flood in Texas that had landed several days prior. As usual, Yvonne chose her favorite acrylic paint colors of pale pastel yellows, light blues, light purple and pinks. In her painting, big streaks of rain slash down from the sky; one could actually see their force, in spite of the transparent colors. The smallish brown structures she painted seem to be cottage houses, though they are fully immersed in the pink, white, blue, and brown water. When we addressed the participants' paintings with media coverage of the natural disaster, I made a comment to Yvonne, who never complains about her devastating disease, maintaining a "stiff upper lip." I said she had portrayed this destructive event very powerfully, but that I thought the cottages being submerged in the water might also speak to her being flooded psychologically by never-ending surgeries, intense pain, feeding tube care and the combination of side effects of her cancer as well as its treatments. She had endured many surgeries and the

radiation therapy, all of which stopped her cancer but also resulted in devastating secondary health issues. While Yvonne consciously set out to illustrate the Texas flood very skillfully, unconsciously, what emerged was her
strong, overwhelming and exhausting feelings of being flooded and nearly
drowning caused by never-ending suffering, pain and self-care that left her
unable to drive, reliant on a walker and unable to eat real food. The pastel colors masked the urgency of her personal suffering on the one hand,
but their transparency—as all colors were mixed with the color white—also
illustrated an acute vulnerability that I associate (but did not verbalize)
with mourning. This interpretation also helped Yvonne's fellow artists in
the group to be more empathic towards her, as it simultaneously opened up
Yvonne's ability to share the many severe, life-threatening symptoms she
concealed and revealed the psychological burden of the effort that it took
her to keep her composure.

Winnicott compares verbal interpretation in a psychoanalytic frame of
reference to a form of mothering, to the ability to identify with the patient
and try to meet their needs verbally, preverbally or nonverbally (Phillips,
1988). The interpretive work that allows the therapist to identify with the
patient communicates maternal care, and only then can the therapeutic setting offer personal growth and lead to better mental health for the patient.

Yvonne's beautiful, sensitive and nearly transparent colors in her painting
of the flood also reminded me of the white, long handsewn simple cotton
gowns that Jews wrap their dead relatives in before they inter them in the
ground or in a simple wood casket for burial. Totally immersed in her present state of intolerable physical crisis, Yvonne unconsciously expressed the
traumatized affective, mental and somatic state she was unable to verbalize,
making it possible for all of us in the support group to empathize with her
suffering and with her unknown future, and with the proximity of a funeral
and death. Having created this obliquely meaningful painting within a creative secure environment, within the transitional space of the Healing Arts
group, Yvonne explored her creative omnipotence that came from within,
becoming proud of her artistic abilities and changing her internal reality of
suffering at that moment into one of mastery in art. Once upright, leaning
on her walker, Yvonne told me that "that was a very meaningful group experience," as if she had just risen from a session on the psychoanalytic couch.

Ogden writes that Winnicott's psychoanalytic method "has in its central
concern the expansion of the capacity of the analyst and patient to create 'a
place to live' in an area of experiencing what lies between reality and fantasy" (Ogden, 1997, pp. 120–121). It is the potential space between the mind
of the art-psychotherapist and that of the patient that invites improvisation,
imagination and exploration. This intersubjective but personal space is not
limited to creative free associations: it also allows us to open up our minds
and freedom of thought in order to discover our creative abilities and play
while addressing difficult issues such as loss and mourning. We can capture

on the canvas the working through of what was missing in our childhood, in conjunction with group members and the art therapist. Art psychotherapy fosters playing together (Phillips, 1988). It invites co-association, and thinking together in our co-creativity, even though we may fall away sometimes to be alone in our reverie, we remain in the presence of the art-psychotherapist, mother or group members (Wildloecher, 2003). Over the course of all this, we can invent images, forms and colors in an attempt towards symbol formation and psychological transformation.

With Winnicott's transitional and potential space, he offers us a therapeutic safe zone that can become a place for creative reparation. As Wildloecher puts it: "Winnicott's [therapeutic technique] formed a dialectical structure that lies at the very foundations of the mental apparatus" (Wildloecher, 2013 [2006]/2012, p. 244). Winnicott's "mental apparatus," the transitional space as applied to art psychotherapy, is a place to play and live in, exploring our personal reality while inviting play and fantasy, in order to become more sensitive and insightful and content as people, in spite of cancer. The integrative power of art making as a form of self-repair allows us to become whole in spite of a potentially life-threatening illness and its often devastating somatic and psychic suffering.

Creative play opens up the unconscious, reaching for our inner visual archive and leaving a record of impressions and accidental traces. It is not unlike Freud's description in 1925 of the notes on the "Mystic Writing Pad": Freud saw *der Wunderblock* as a metaphor for the self and the perception of time. "It is as though the unconscious stretches out feelers through the preconscious towards the external world and hastily withdraws them, as soon as they have sampled the excitations coming from them," writes Freud (1925, p. 231). Here, the pad is the art-psychoanalytic setting, the studio, the attention of the art therapist, and group members, in that they define the potential space with traces from the present and the past (Green, 2013, pp. 183–204). The different surfaces of the Mystic Writing Pad are interrelated between conscious and unconscious memory traces, yet remain parts of one system. So does the artist retrieve images linked to memories that form her pictorial archive, while also using urgent and significant personal material from the present to mold their content with the help of free associations, color and form (Dreifuss-Kattan, 1986, pp. 15–16).

Zizi Raymond said about her experience in the Cancer and Creativity group that

> It's hard to get away from the idea that you have cancer. We are making art in an Oncology office. When you are there, you are in the cancer part of your life. I have metastatic cancer. I can't get away from it anyway.

Metastatic cancer is a life-threatening disease, as cancer cells spill to other organs or into the bloodstream and become more difficult to destroy or contain with traditional cancer treatments (Figure 2.2).

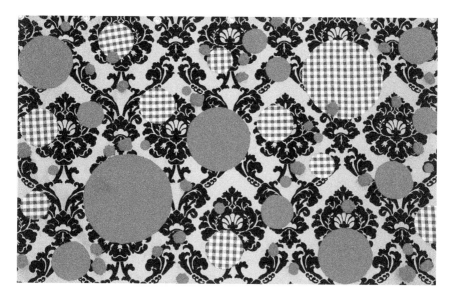

Figure 2.2 Zizi Raymond, "Blood Production," 2010, Silk, Felt, and Gingham Fabric.

In her fabric mural *Blood Production* (2010), Zizi used felt and gingham fabric on silk. "Here in my fabric mural the cancer cells are multiplying and dividing in the bloodstream." We might call *Blood Production* a fabric mural or big blanket: the red cancer cells created with red felt seem to multiply, from very small circles to medium and big red cells, stitched together with white and black-checkered smaller circles. The pattern is laid out beautifully and with great care on a big silk fabric with a gold and black background. The fabric is smooth to the touch and looks more elegant and playful than menacing. The circular forms of blood cells of Zizi's fabric collage are beautifully balanced, their equilibrium communicating a unifying, tranquil impression to the viewer at odds with the aggravated symptoms the collage illustrates. *Blood Production* reminded me of the transitional object, remembering that for Winnicott it is a blanket, teddy bear or any soft comforting object that the baby finds, when she gets ready to separate from mother but still wants to be connected, easing the temporary separation. Zizi was always very deliberate in her choices of materials and varied use of forms. Using soft, elegant fabric with its comfortable touch was a good medium for her as her cancer metastasized and the threat of separation started to loom. In fearful times we reach into our personal archives of the past to search for comfort in the present. The soft blanket of infancy endures as a beautiful and comforting wall hanging, though it gains a rather menacing message.

Psychological self-repair through art making when confronted with cancer might also, therefore, speak to the unconscious wish that the finished artwork would reinstate the physical balance in the body itself that was destroyed by cancer and its treatment. The search for the artistic form is the search for an intact body as well as the flourishing of the wish to rediscover one's invulnerable creative self, which in spite of illness can be vibrant, alive and still growing. There the artist rediscovers a primary narcissistic balance that can be achieved through the unity of the artistic form once finished and the comforting aspect of being-with-oneself in the creative process. The beautiful composition of the fabric mural stands in for, and has nurtured, the wish for a coherent psychic integration.

This transitional object found in the outside world is the child's first possession—thumb, blanket, teddy bear—that is invested with the products of subjectivity. Endowing the transitional object with the content of his or her inner world, the child or adult can create an illusionary connection with the early experience of a protecting mother or force. The transitional object, for Winnicott, is vital to the development of a real self-separate from them. Because it is both created by the infant or toddler (or artist) and is provided by the world outside their subjectivity, it is the child's first experience of "not-me," as an object that can be created as "mine." It is, in a way, the first defensive reaction to loss, the loss of the mother in its earliest form in the infant's life, and a way to negotiate the potential losses of the cancer patient. The blanket for the infant—or the artwork for the artist—allows them to both tolerate the loss and to fashion a new experience and/or an object to work with the loss and so create continuity. The transitional object is an actual, material object, as we have seen in Zizi's fabric collage, and it endures in the external world, to be lost and rediscovered again. Every new artwork secures the connection to an internal reality and at the same time manages its continuity with outside reality. The fabric mural or the small sculpture functions as a talisman to ward off anxieties and the fear of death and to exist after death, securing an immortality for its maker (Dreifuss-Kattan, 1990).

The fear of death from cancer is often, psychoanalytically, an unconscious fear of being overtaken by bad internal objects, realized by tumors or metastasis, and in Zizi's case by cancerous blood cells that ultimately consume their victims. This race against the slow process of physical destruction is thus counteracted by the artist's ego ideal which redirects her focus on art making and connecting to good, creative internal objects; for Zizi this was her loving grandmother. Through exhibiting her art to the public and being recognized within the group of fellow cancer-travellers, Zizi satisfied her omnipotent narcissistic and psychic pleasure, opposing the malignant internal process symbolized by the cancerous tumors. Identifying with the ego ideal, a productive artist can then relieve fears and partly suspend the threatening reality around her (Meerwein, 1989).

Practicing artists are perhaps better equipped to use their creativity in an attempt to express and project their feelings, longings and physical experience onto a sculpture or canvas. They are used to communicating with their viewers through forms and colors and can project their physical status or their feelings in spite of cancer, strengthening their sense of self-love and mastery in spite of a potentially life-threatening disease. Even without being a professional artist, being creative in the face of cancer, can satisfy omnipotent and narcissistic needs that were so badly damaged by the destructive progress of the disease and its often devastating treatments. Thoughts of equilibrium or restoration of the self can then be reconsidered anew (Dreifuss-Kattan, 1990).

Force Fed (2009) is another sculpture that Zizi created during this time period, at a low point of enjoyment of her own body and her own self. She started to lose weight and did not feel like eating much. "This piece is about eating as a chore," she writes. "I had it before I had to force myself to eat following my whole brain radiation. It foretold what I would experience later" (Raymond, 2010). This sculpture is made with 12 lightweight plastic spoons with globs of hardened uncolored grey clay in each one. A little earlier Zizi had created another piece called *Fork Box* (2008). Delicate cocktail forks bristle menacingly. "Eating is difficult," writes Zizi in the catalogue of her exhibition. The curt, exasperated comment speaks to years of living with breast cancer treatments. Now she had become more vulnerable and wanted nothing to go down her throat any longer. Zizi was disgusted, at that moment, with hospitalizations, surgeries and radiation. She soldiered on soon thereafter, meeting the next difficult phase of her cancer (Figure 2.3).

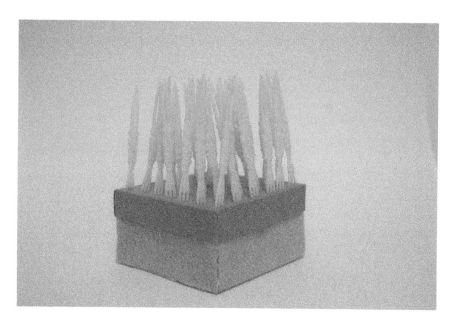

Figure 2.3 Zizi Raymond, "Fork Box," 2008, Cardboard Box, Acryl Paint and Plastic Forks.

Zizi's vitrine box, with its old medical textbook slides of cutup body parts, *Blood Production, Force Fed* and *Fork Box* all document the breakdown of her body and the suffering she felt as even basic functions like swallowing began to halt. By the time I got to know this artist-patient, cancer had spread to many of her organs, and its effects radiated throughout her way of life. In spite of her state, Zizi Raymond never came late to the art group, and she always stayed to the end. One time, she arrived after a horrific session of whole brain radiation, another time after brain laser surgery. After most group sessions, she returned to her studio and continued to draw and paint. Zizi's art addresses and mourns her many losses: the loss of her physical endurance, loss of her appetite, loss of her depth of vision and eventually the loss of her very treasured independence. Indeed, on a pragmatic level, Zizi had to find new, less physically demanding media than those she preferred when she was strong and healthy, and was building, among other things, large, solid metal sculptures. More metaphorically, using scissors for cutting out the round fabric pieces for *Blood Production*, or an Exacto knife for her paper collages, allowed this artist to channel and express physically some of the destructive and aggressive aspects of this malignant process, such as the invasion of destructive cancerous cells. As her art made the somatic realm its content, however, it transformed it in an aesthetic realm that redeemed it and enabled her perseverance. Losses like those Zizi endured can result in a strong desire to reconnect with and reconstruct the early supportive primary object, a parent or grandparent; yet, as in her case, they also instill the longing for a new artistic Gestalt, its innovative technical solutions and aesthetic form an attempt for psychological reparation and the preparation for more separation and its attendant mourning.

At its most idealistic, aesthetic form is the mediating factor between what is experienced as inside and as outside, and this ideal is what seems to guarantee the wish of the patient to inhabit her art, to take on the unity of its composition. Such an afterlife, for Zizi, is maintained in this soft fabric mural produced while her illness progressed, which, due to this softness and likeness to Winnicott's prototypical transitional object, becomes the mediating symbol of togetherness and separation and of dying and immortality. Indeed, the mediating power of the aesthetic bridges not only Zizi's interior and exterior realities, but the artist and the spectator. Like a transitional object here as well, the collage or sculpture is marking the borderland where it seems that self and other are eliminated as they become dialectically united. The viewers are seduced by the aesthetic pleasure of form and color, a sort of unconscious reliving or empathizing, a form of identification that allows us to touch upon our own early separations and successful experience of mourning from the past, and even take Zizi's own wish for reintegration seriously in the form of her work, since that reintegration becomes an undeniable emotional reality for us as spectators.

Ultimately, it is the search for an aesthetic form and a reliable relationship—as well as the unconscious wish for the original unity between mother and child—that animates the art making of the cancer patient. When we address mourning and mortality through creative means, the artist often achieves a feeling of psychological integration, as the art embodies a profound personal experience for the artist and all of the group members and the public that views the art. "It addresses the juncture of life and death with which we all can identify" (Dreifuss-Kattan, 1990, p. 149). Artistic and formalistic talent can provide the artist with cancer some emotional detachment in negotiating overwhelming feelings, and thus help their viewers to identify with the enduring sense of wholeness and with the good internal object. Like the transitional object that was used in early life as the symbol for the absent mother, Zizi's craftsmanship in making her fabric collage invests the cancerous blood cells with the capacity to be beautiful (Dreifuss-Kattan, 1990, p. 130). This creative tapestry becomes a "transformational object," as it is "transforming and redefining the boundaries of subjectivity and culture, including the boundaries between conscious and unconscious experience and knowledge" (Schwab, 2010, p. 7) Art making, and sharing artwork with a group or with public viewership, converts the artist with cancer's very private experience of loss and mourning into a more universal one. Creative expression counterbalances the many losses connected to cancer with a love for life, allowing the patient to identify with the good breast, and the good inner object, giving new life through new material, forms and color.

Note

1   Milner's first interest was also in Jungian analytical theories and Eastern philosophies. Her first book, *A Life of One's Own* (1936), was published under the name Joanna Field to great acclaim, and was reviewed by W.H. Auden. Another important book is *The Hands of the Living God*, which uses the drawings and doodles of her psychotic patient as an integral part of several years of psychoanalytic treatment. The book was informed by Milner's own love for art, as she was an excellent painter herself.

References

Derrida, J. (1995). *Archive Fever: A Freudian Impression* (E. Prenowitz, Trans.). Chicago, IL: The University of Chicago Press.

Dreifus-Kattan, E. (1986) *Praxis der klinischen Kunst Therapie Pracice of Clinical Art Therapy*. Stuttgard, Toronto: Verlag Hans Huber Bern.

Dreifuss-Kattan, E. (1990) *Cancer Stories: Creativity and Self-Repair*. Hillsdale NJ: The Analytic Press.

Farley, L. (2013). Squiggle Evidence: The Child, the Canvas, and the 'Negative Labor' of History. In J. Abram (Ed.), *Donald Winnicott Today* (pp. 418–452). London: Routledge.

Freud, S. (1914). Totem and Taboo. In A. Richards (Ed.), *The Standard Edition of the Complete Psychological Works of Sigmund Freud: Totem and Taboo and Other Works* (Vol. 13) (J. Strachey, Trans.) (pp. 211–236). London: The Hogarth Press and the Institute of Psychoanalysis.

Field, J. [Marion Milner] (1936/1981). *A Life of One's Own*. New York: Putnam.

Green, A. (2013). Potential Space in Psychoanalysis: The Object in the Setting. In J. Abram (Ed.), *Donald Winnicott Today* (pp. 183–204). London: Routledge.

Langer, S. (1953). *Feeling and Form*. New York: Charles Scribner's Sons.

Meerwein, F. (1989). Zeiterleben im psychoanalytischen Prozess. *Psychosomatische Medizin u. Psychoanal.*, 2, 156–174.

Milner, M. (1969). *The Hands of the Living God*. New York: International University Press.

Milner, M. (1972–7) (2013). Winnicott: Overlapping Circles and the Two-Way Journey. In J. Abram (Ed.), *Donald Winnicott Today* (pp. 168–182). London: Routledge and the Institude of Psychoanalysis in London.

Odgen, T. (1985). The Mother, the Infant and the Matrix: Interpretations of Aspects of the Works of Donald Winicott. In J. Abram and A. Emma (Ed.), Donald Winnicott Today (pp. 46–72). London: Routledge, and Institute of psychoanalysis.

Ogden, T. (1997). *Reverie and Interpretation*. London: Jason Aronson.

Phillips, A. (1988). *D. W. Winnicott*. Cambridge, MA: Harvard University Press.

Phillips, A. (2017a, October 26). *Conversion Hysteria: Believe It Or Not*. Presentation at the New Center for Psychoanalysis, Santa Monica, CA.

Phillips, A. (2017b, October 28). *Winnicott's Magic: Playing and Reality* and Reality Presentation at the New Center for Psychoanalysis, Santa Monica, CA.

Phillips, A. (2006). *Modern Classic Penguin Freud Reader*. Penguin Modern Classic

Phillips, A. (1998). *On Kissingg, Tickling, and Being Bored: Psychoanalytic Essay on Unexamined Life*.

Raymond, Z. (2009). Works on Paper and Sculpture. Catalogue 2009, Santa Monica CA, Premiere Oncology Foundation.

Schwab, G. (2010). *Haunting Legacies: Violent Histories and Transgenerational Trauma*. New York: Columbia University Press.

Schwab, G. (2012). *Imaginary Ethnographies: Literature, Culture and Subjectivity*. New York: Columbia University Press.

Wildloecher, D. (2006) 2012. Winnicott and the Acquisition of a Freedom of Thought. In J. Abram (Ed.), *Donald Winnicott Today* (pp. 235–249). London: Routledge.

Winnicott, D. W. (1971). *Playing and Reality*. London: Tavistock.

Chapter 3

One in eight

Fighting breast cancer with embroidery and knitting

Christine Carey and Suzanne Isken

Artist: Christine Carey

When I created my embroidered handkerchiefs and knitted my cupcakes inspired by the "Cancer and Creativity" group I participated in, it was probably the first time in my life that I had created something without specific use in mind.

There were no books in my house when I was growing up. No paper, no paints. The first time I ever saw paint and paper is when I went to school at four and a half. I was told at the age of five by my kindergarten teacher that I had no talent for painting. They had easels with big pieces of paper and poster paint. I had never seen anything like that before. We had to draw a house. So I drew a house but my teacher, who was not an art teacher, told me it didn't look like a house. She told me to go and stand in the playground and look at the houses opposite. I was devastated. Maybe that's what taught me "you can't be an artist. You can't even draw a house!"

At the age of 60 I participated in the "Cancer and Creativity" group and found out that I still can't draw. However, with Esther's help, I learned to express myself in many other creative media, like cut paper and sewing clothing and costumes for children and grandchildren. I came to the realization that I have been creating art and crafts in different forms all my life. Knitting and embroidery have always been therapeutic and calming activities for me. The delicate vintage fabrics and the thin tracery of embroidery are in direct contrast to the extensive physical and psychological traumas my body and mind suffered during my cancer journey. I was satisfied by the pleasure these items gave to the recipients and the recognition I received.

I always feel peaceful and calm when creating something. When I was a child "making" was, it seemed, the only activity I was good at and that I also enjoyed. I enjoyed being alone with myself.

My creations for family and friends almost always contain humor, sometimes dark, sometimes not. As my granddaughter remarked recently: "Grandma, you're weird, but in a good way." My colorful embroideries, although serious in theme, are also funny.

Did knitting put the cancer experience behind me? By the time I finished these doilies, I did think that I had put the cancer behind me. However, actively creating these images and revisiting that traumatic time and creating something from this most difficult time period, at first just for me, felt satisfying, worthwhile and healing.

I first started to knit the cupcakes, and shortly after the embroideries. My mother had taught me to knit when I was six years old; even so, she preferred her sewing machine. I remember the first thing I ever created was a rabbit, sewn from pieces of a dress that belonged to my mother. I can still see it today; it was an off-white bouclé material that I had cut out on the dining room table, while cutting the tablecloth below as well. My mother was not happy!

My childhood friend next door, Christine, had a Chinese grandmother. Her grandfather was a missionary and had married a woman there, and she came to live with my friend's family. She was very clever and talented. She taught us to cook and to smock. I always remember smocking these little dresses we made. I was about 10 or 11 then. We were being groomed to be good housewives. I grew up in a place called Shefferton in England, next door to the Shefferton film studios. It was a small town; we later moved to a small house on the River Thames when I was about six.

By the time I was 12, I was a very competent knitter and sewer. I knitted sweaters. I was always making things—little doll beds out of boxes that had contained dates. We also spent a lot of time on the River Thames messing about in boats and nearly drowning.

We had a local knitting shop run by a very kind lady who would help me if I ever ran into a problem because my mum was only a very basic knitter. I used to buy the wool from her, often brown and cream because those were my favorite colors to wear. I even tailored my own clothes as a girl, and as I got older I had to sew my own clothes because I couldn't afford to buy them. I used to go to the markets in London and buy fabric from the traders there, traders called barrow boys because they sold off a wheelbarrow. I also sewed and went to the traders because of her creative grandma.

I was pretty much a loner as a child. I spent a lot of time alone in my bedroom making things and painting. I got married very young. I wanted to go to art school, but that wasn't available to me because my parents thought I should learn to type. So the only opportunity I had was to go to Pittman's Secretarial College, which was a nightmare. I only stayed a year and then I left home at age 17 and went to live in Cornwall with the hippies.

I had my first child at 20. I continued to make my own clothes and my kids' clothes, and even my husband's clothes. My creativity took a more practical turn then, and I never considered what I created as art. I still have a problem with calling myself an artist. I remember knitting Erin/Aaron's, my kids', sweaters. I oiled the wool to make it waterproof.

I made amazing patterns but I never considered myself clever. It was just something I did. I did consider it fun while I was doing it. I liked creating it. I'm not very good at identifying feelings about things. It was a way of life for me.

In the 1960s I remember making loads of miniskirts and hot pants. When I had my first child, I made my own nighties. They didn't give you a hospital gown in those days. I made a short "Mong" that was very popular at the time out of flimsy beige-white fabric, and then a long robe to go over it. I remember the doctors commenting on it. It was very sixties. Of course, I made most of the kids' clothes and their costumes for school plays. I guess I did like doing it—otherwise I wouldn't have done it, would I? It was always an outlet for me because I would get lost in it. I don't really ever remember being terribly happy, but I was born on a Wednesday. You know, "Wednesday's child is full of woe." My mother wasn't a very happy person either—I guess that might have something to do with it. I think she always had slight depression, which I have fought with too. I always think of myself as a house that might have dry rot—it looks fine but it might be falling apart (Figures 3.1 and 3.2).

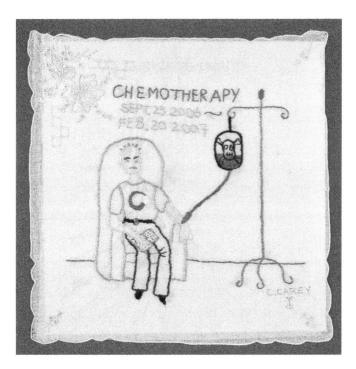

Figure 3.1 Christine Carey, "Chemotherapy," 2012, Embroidery on Vintage Handkerchief.

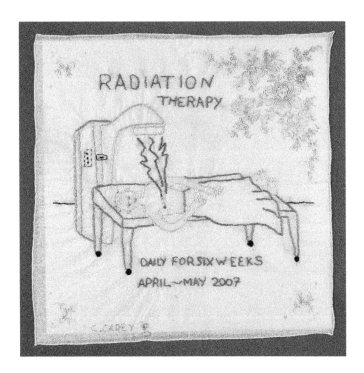

Figure 3.2 Christine Carey, "Radiation Therapy," 2012, Embroidery on Vintage Handkerchief.

When I was diagnosed with breast cancer, I handled it like I've handled everything all my life, with one foot in front of the other. This is what you have to do. I was lucky—I had family and I had friends and a lot of support. I just took it a day at a time and got through. I can't say I was ever frightened. I didn't like all the surgeries, but I never thought I would die. This contradicts what I've already told you about myself, but I think I was always able to see a more positive side while going through my cancer experience.

When I came to the "Cancer and Creativity" group, it was three or four years after diagnosis. I had worked in an often very creative environment for a publisher that made pop-up books. I was not a paper engineer, but I was the production manager and surrounded by creativity. That was inspiring and I did make things, but nothing I ever kept.

Esther, the leader of the "Cancer and Creativity" group mentioned an art show, which I'd never even considered before I put more time and effort into my creations. This group experience was something I'd never experienced,

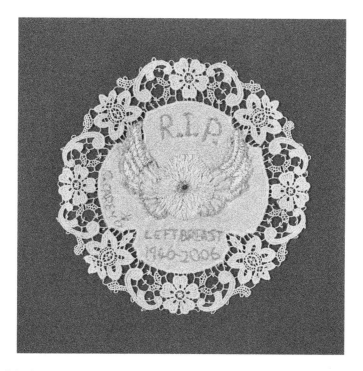

Figure 3.3 Christine Carey, "R.I.P.," 2012, Embroidery on Vintage Handkerchief.

as I'd always created alone. I quite like being alone and doing stuff. It's sort of a selfish thing. I don't have to consider anybody else. I've been looking after people all my life (Figure 3.3).

The first piece I stitched was on a doily, the round one that said: "Rest In Peace." It was embroidery of a breast. That's what started it. I'd had these vintage handkerchiefs for a long time, but what do you do with them? You don't use them as hankies, do you? So I thought, oh, that'll be good, I'll use those. And then it just started. I broke the story down into the mastectomy, the chemo and so on. So that's how it came about. I started out sketching it first and then I did the embroidery just looking at the sketch on the paper.

I found a knitting pattern for a cupcake, and then used the idea to make my own pattern. One in eight women will have cancer in their lifetime, so I decided to knit eight cupcakes and one of them would have cancer. I also made paper cupcake holders out of small paper doilies and shaped them with Mod Podge to make them stiff. People still look at them on the cupcake tray in my home and wonder at first if they're real (Figure 3.4).

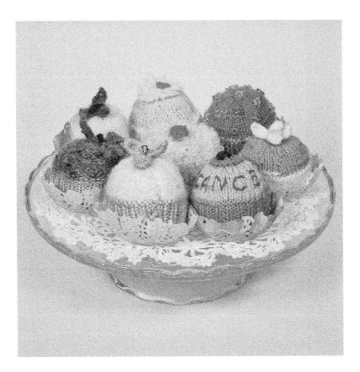

Figure 3.4 Christine Carey, "Mastectomy," 2012, Embroidery on Vintage Handkerchief.

How the craft practices of embroidery and knitting became forms of artistic expression

Suzanne Isken

Craft as we know it today emerged as a political force to reunite the maker with their humanity. The Studio Craft Movement reconnected craft work with meaning, pride and personal identity at a time when mechanization and urbanization threatened to replace the human hand. It was born in the late 1880s in England and developed to free artisans from the necessity of creating objects for functional purpose alone. The British Studio Craft Movement represented a push toward reuniting craft with the pleasure of creative work. William Morris (1834–1896), a leader of the British Arts and Crafts Movement, took up embroidery himself in 1855, in defiance of the notion that manual labor was unsuitable for a gentleman.

In 1984, art historian Rozsika Parker first published her research on the history of embroidery and its relationship to the status of women in *The Subversive Stitch: Embroidery and the Making of the Feminine.* Parker used diaries, women's magazines, letters, novels and works of art to examine how the separation of the craft of embroidery from the category of fine arts came to be typical of the denigration of women's work, even as embroidery still provided women with a source of creativity and community. Historically, an education in the textile arts meant reproducing traditional design patterns. In the 1940s, a debate emerged in the textile arts world between the conservatism of traditional forms and the Bauhaus ideology of creating new, original forms from a process of experimentation, associated with younger artists like Anni Albers and Black Mountain College. These artists broke from the restrictions of the past and invented new means of expression. Following the Second World War, their contemporary art theory gained popularity among the infusion of returning students flooding art and technical schools on the G.I. bill, who melded traditional functional arts with a burgeoning abstract art movement. Media-specific art practices such as textiles, ceramics, glass and metalworking were liberated from their functional histories and embraced by the fine arts world as another means of abstract composition. Woven works and needlework came off the loom to liberate themselves from traditional materials and enter the third dimension.

As abstraction became an increasingly limiting means of self-expression, a new generation of artists like Robert Rauschenberg embraced readymade quilts, decorative patterns and craft media as a means of making art more accessible by infusing it with "real life." Materials were soon chosen more for their sociopolitical associations than their material properties. In the early 1970s women artists addressed issues of gender and domestic space by embracing art forms associated with women's work, including needle arts and ceramic painting. Remembering Parker's research, these domestic crafts opened an avenue for making political statements about their exclusion from the art market. Feminist artists including Judy Chicago, Miriam Shapiro and Joyce Scott reignited the interest in textile arts by using techniques of sewing, embroidery and beading. These artists, trained primarily as painters and sculptors, had long rejected domestic arts because of their association with the confined lives of their own mothers and grandmothers. Eager to create a dialectic that might negate the gigantic, imposing steel sculptures of male artists such as Richard Serra, feminist artists such as Miriam Shapiro championed the soft sculpture, the handmade, the stitched and sewn. In embracing arts made in the domestic sphere, these artists were not so much celebrating domesticity as standing in solidarity with the women who found time to make art between the long hours spent cooking, clearing and caring for a family.

Christine Carey's embroidery in the context of craft

Although this feminist dialectic seems open to the charge of simply appropriating women's craft history, the materials and making processes of that history serve as metaphors and symbols that communicate complex meaning. Miriam Shapiro, like Christine Carey, chose the handkerchief as an art making material. She reported: "Besides being interested in their aesthetics, handkerchiefs were also the repository of oceans of tears and curiously enough messages from the body" (Bradly, Apelhof, & Shapiro, 1980, pp. 47–48). Handkerchiefs are objects of comfort or relief when held close to the body. Carey recognized the fragility of the antique handkerchief, too precious to use for blowing your nose. Vintage cloth has been used by artists to represent memory, history and a link with sentimentality. Artists such as Betye Saar have spoken about their use of found fabrics as a means of associating with domesticity, history and female labor. Sewing connotes repair, healing and renewal. A new movement of art as mending has social, political and environmental agendas behind its popularity. Embroidery has been particularly singled out as a means of making that does not introduce more objects into a world that has too many material goods already.

The metaphor of sewing takes on additional meaning in Christine Carey's embroidered work titled *Mastectomy, 2012*. Here Carey actually pierces the thin surface of the cloth, a form of violence to an object held so long as a precious keepsake. Her stitches also decorate and add new value and meaning, however. Creating the embroidery to tell the story of her breast cancer, Carey evokes a narrative that is personal, feminine and associated with a particular point in time. She aligns herself here with the more recent work of artist Jenny Hart who founded Sublime Stitching. Hart's motto is "This ain't your gramma's embroidery." Hart connects with contemporary culture through embroidering tattooed portraits of legendary figures, for instance.

Christine Carey's work in the context of knitted craft

Through her knitted work *One in Eight* (2012), Carey joined a growing movement of craftivists who have married their social and political concerns with the act of knitting and embroidering. The second-wave feminists reminded us that the personal is political. As Carey embraces knitting to publicize the astonishing statistic that one out or every eight women will be diagnosed with breast cancer, she joins the ranks of artists like Cat Mazza, Lisa Auerbach and Margarita Cabrera who sew, knit and embroider works about war, the environment and the plight of immigrants from Mexico. Carey's eight cupcake breasts can be interpreted both as a warning that living life as a female can be dangerous to your health or an admonition to us all that you can put a man on the moon but you cannot stop one in eight women from getting breast cancer. Her brilliant metaphor recalls every Victoria Secret advertisement that dressed up breasts in pink lace and presented them for consumption (Figure 3.5).

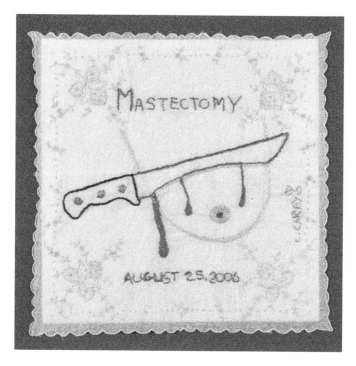

Figure 3.5 Christine Carey, "One in Eight," 2012, Knitting Wool and Paper.

Through the activities of activist knitting groups, knitting has become "a radical alternative to the commodification of all aspects of life" (Robertson, 2011, p. 18). Furthermore, some knitters have taken to the streets to challenge the portrayal of activists as violent and destructive. By championing their power through knitting and protest, women have found a voice. Recently, we have seen hundreds of women marching internationally in knitted pink Pussyhats with cat ears, a reference to Donald Trump's vulgar statements about grabbing women's genitals. The women who knit the hats described them as a physical manifestation of their anger toward the president-elect's statements about women, minorities and the disabled (Mehta, 2017).

Craft and the healing arts

In choosing knitting as a medium for expressing her experience with breast cancer, Carey not only recalls her own creative history and the history of female creativity but also refers to a means of creative coping that has been widely practiced and acknowledged by makers of all levels of skill. The craft community understands and embraces the importance of making for surviving tragedy. Grounded in Progressive Era and Arts and Crafts Movement social ideals, the notion that engaging a patient's mind and body shortened convalescence, and the belief that disabled persons could function in their communities despite physical roadblocks informed General John J. Pershing's order to teach needlework to recovering soldiers who were wounded during WWI. In 1941, Major General Frederick H. Osborn, brother of American Craft Council founder Aileen Osborn Webb, was appointed chairman of the War Department Committee on Education, Recreation and Community Service to help raise "morale" among soldiers and veterans. He helped institute arts and crafts programs in military camps, which made craft accessible to thousands of soldiers.

Contemporary craft advocates would not have been surprised to learn the findings of a study at Otago University, New Zealand. A total of 658 students were asked to keep diaries of their experiences and emotional states over 13 days; the study found that people who participated in arts and crafts feel happier, calmer and more energetic the next day. A Daily Mail report of the study published in November 2016 in the Journal of Positive Psychology was widely circulated by artists following the last US presidential election (Ough, 2016).

Coincidently, an international organization called Knitted Knockers sprang up in 2007 to knit prosthetic breasts (not unlike the pattern Carey uses for her cupcake breasts) for women who have had mastectomies. Knitted Knockers has grown into a worldwide organization called Knitted Knockers Charities, a 501c3 public charity. The website www.KnittedKnockersUSA. org and www.knittedknockers.org provide knitting patterns, knitting tips and information on approved yarns. In the United States, there are groups in Arizona, Arkansas, California, Florida, Georgia, Idaho, Illinois, Indiana, New York, Maryland, Michigan, Minnesota, Ohio, Pennsylvania, Texas, Tennessee, Washington, Wisconsin plus Knitted Knockers UK, Knitted Knockers Australia, Knitted Knockers South Africa and Knitted Knockers Alberta. They join groups in Mexico, Germany and Finland that are making, donating and/or distributing knitted knockers in their local areas.

Pictures

1   Christine Carey: One In Eight: One in Eight Women Will Be Diagnosed with Breast Cancer in the USA 2012, Knitting wool, ceramic, paper
2   Mastectomy: 2012 Embroidery on Vintage Handkerchief, 16″ × 16″
3   Chemotherapy: 2012 Embroidery on Vintage Handkerchief, 16″ × 164″
4   Radiation: 2012 Embroidery on Vintage Handkerchief, 16″ × 16″
5   Reconstruction: 2011 Embroidery on Vintage Handkerchief, 16″ × 16″
6   R.I.P. 2012 Embroidery on Vintage Handkerchief, 16″ × 16″

References

Bell, N. (2012). *40 Under 40 Craft Futures.* Washington, DC: Renwick Gallery Smithsonian American Art Museum.

Bradly, P., Apelhof, R.A., and Shapiro, M. (1980). Excerpts from Interviews with Miriam Shapiro. Interview. In T. Gouma-Peterson (Ed.), *Miriam Shapiro: A Retrospective, 1953–1980* (pp. 47–48). Wooster, OH: College of Wooster.

Koplos, J. and Metcalf, B. (2010). *Makers: A History of American Studio Craft.* Chapel Hill: University of North Carolina Press.

Mehta, S. (2017, January 15). How These Los Angeles-Born Pink Hats Became a Worldwide Symbol of the Anti-Trump Women's March. *Los Angeles Times.* Retrieved from www.latimes.com/politics/la-pol-ca-pink-hats-womens-march-20170115story.html.

Ough, T. (2016, November 25). Knitting, Crocheting and Jam-Making Improve Mental Health, Study Finds. *Daily Telegraph.* Retrieved from www.telegraph.co.uk/news/2016/11/25/knitting-crocheting-jam-making-improve-mental-health-study-finds/.

Parker, R. (2010). *The Subversive Stitch: Embroidery and the Making of the Feminine* (2nd ed.). London: I.B.Tauris.

Robertson, K. (2011). Rebellious Doilies and Subversive Stitches: Writing a Craftivist History. In M.E. Buszek (Ed.), *Extra/Ordinary Craft and Contemporary Art* (pp. 108–109). Durham, NC: Duke University Press.

Chapter 4

Cutting, pasting and piercing

A memoir of healing

Corinne Lightweaver

Coming to terms with the physical changes of midlife took on new meaning for me when I was diagnosed with breast cancer. Should I remove only the diseased breast or take both to decrease future risks? I chose to have both removed and opted for reconstruction. The seven-month period of wearing expanders—balloons of saline—under the skin to stretch it in preparation for the implants was grueling. I had to juggle the pain, the foreign objects in my body and the new borders of my femininity and sexuality. I tried to joke about it to ease the impact, referring to my "margarine-tub breasts" and "bionic boobs" and to my choice of a bilateral mastectomy as "sanity" versus "vanity." But beyond humor and humility, the most empowering ally on my journey to healing was returning to the art studio. Making art allowed me to access unconscious and uncomfortable feelings about my breast cancer. Four years earlier I had ceased making art while battling lymphoma. Ultimately, and ironically, breast cancer restored my vitality as an artist.

During the six months following my diagnosis of breast cancer and immediate bilateral mastectomy in 2007, friends and family had puzzled me with comments about how "calm" and "courageous" I was. I felt serenity on the surface, but until I turned to art for healing, I had no idea of a contrast between my behavior and anything transpiring beneath it. As I worked with art materials and let my unconscious lead the way, I encountered the complicated mix of horror and wonder that is at the core of surviving breast cancer.

As often happens to patients, my diagnosis was unexpected—an irregular mammogram. A biopsy. Then, wham. A few days before my daughter's first day of kindergarten, I received the news, along with the verdict from the surgeon that I should have surgery within three weeks. A second opinion confirmed the first. Quick decisions required quick thinking. There wasn't much time. The oncological surgeon expressed a low opinion of one of two plastic surgeons my insurance plan covered. My wife, my mother and I went to see the doctor that the oncological surgeon deemed acceptable. When we talked with him, however, he focused, enthusiastically, on enhancing the size of my breasts rather than repairing my body. We saw the photos of his work. We cried. My wife campaigned for another surgeon.

We selected an outside plastic surgeon who worked alongside the oncological surgeon during the first surgery. But as my wife sought insurance coverage for our plastic surgeon, the oncology surgeon denied she had indicated a negative opinion and my longtime general physician backed her.

Thus, the workings of a cold bureaucracy unfolded seemingly in indifference to the intimate details of my body. There was no time to wait for genetic testing results. I weighed my previous diagnosis of lymphoma, my paternal Ashkenazi Jewish family's history of breast cancer and my wish to be alive to parent my daughter—and chose to have both breasts removed immediately. After the bilateral mastectomy, I received news that I have the BRCA-2 gene, meaning I have a higher risk for both breast cancer and ovarian cancer than the general population. Further testing revealed surprising results. My father did not carry the BRCA-2 gene, as expected, because of his Ashkenazi Jewish heritage; it had been my mother, who had no history of cancer in her family.

In the weeks before and after the surgery, I had no time to dwell on feelings. Decisions needed to be made not only about my surgery but also about my daughter's care and my wife's work schedule. Shortly after the surgery, my wife launched an epic battle with the insurance company over coverage of my preferred plastic surgeon. That battle, unexpectedly, also tore us apart. She dealt with facts and figures, policies and protocols, and did it well. But I missed her emotional support, and we couldn't seem to bridge the gap. Creating art about my experience crucially not only helped me but also helped my wife understand the feelings that either I was not able to communicate or she was not able to hear. Art helped me to talk to her and to find myself.

Often what was transmitted to paper, canvas or shaped in a three-dimensional creation was *breaking news* to me. In art therapy, when I gave my unconscious the sacred space to speak, it delivered unprecedented messages. The information could give voice to an unspoken emotion or solve a knotty problem. It could express numbness, joy, gratitude, anger, despair or playfulness. It could be blatantly clear or it could be in the form of a coded message. Sometimes my art therapist and my fellow artists—the majority of whom were not formally trained—could decode what I did not notice myself.

Diving in

Some artists know exactly what they're going to paint or sculpt and how, but that's not me. Often I have a topic or framework, but how I get to the finished piece and what it's going to look like is always a mystery. Since

I began drawing and painting roughly ten years before my breast cancer diagnosis, my progress had been this unpredictable, and in the art therapy group it remained so. When I am making art amid such uncertainty, it is also often necessary for me to resist the negative voice inside that tells me I'm not a good enough artist and that I don't know what I am doing. I have learned to reply that it can keep on talking, but I'm going to keep painting anyway.

The blank canvas or page can be challenging for many artists. The prompts I received from the art therapist at the beginning of each session were helpful to get going, but I never knew what the outcome of my efforts would be. Often I would follow the prompt and choose one of the suggested materials. Sometimes I also found it helpful to have suggested topics or media to reject so that I could launch in my own direction.

That the art I created in the therapy space evolved into something with wings—something that had a life outside therapy—was a surprise, especially in the beginning. Art created in the therapy space does not have to be "great art" to be effective. But when it stands on its own as a legitimate piece of art, it can bring its creator a wider audience with which to share her message. Art became part of my healing process as it not only allowed me to discover my feelings but it could also evoke an emotional response in others. When my art was exhibited, it was very gratifying to have a visitor tell me "I didn't know it was like that"; or "you expressed something I felt but didn't know how to describe." It turned out that therapeutic art could do more than encompass my personal experience: it led me to interface with viewers and guided my interaction with my fellow patients and survivors in the therapy group.

Finding community

The art therapy space was where I could feel miserable, happy, whatever. All of it was okay. And if I was feeling numb, that was okay too. I created in the art therapy space because that was the task in front of me. Especially in the first year and a half, I didn't know why or what or how.

Whether I was numb or overwhelmed with feelings, making art was a simple way to engage my hands. And eventually my heart and mind. Unlike in my life dealing with cancer, there were no big decisions to be made. Choose ocher or citrine, maroon or vermillion. Grasp coarse burlap, fine brocade or burnished leather. Through cutting, pasting and piecing, I was putting my body and my psyche back together.

I was creating for myself, or, rather, *the process* was for myself. The only expectation was participation—and even that was optional. Many pieces I created were ultimately for process only—it helped that I didn't always have to create "good" art. Each piece taught me something useful about myself, but I didn't have to share every piece outside the therapy room. The option of privacy took the pressure off. It allowed *all* the art I created to serve my therapy.

For most of the time during communal art making, we were engaged in parallel play, creating adjacent to each other but separately and without trying to influence each other. Small talk was not necessary in the art therapy space. It was an eggshell-free zone. I didn't have to worry about shocking my group mates with my cancer stories or trying to protect them from the impact of hearing about my experiences. That constructed permission to be silent, in contrast to my experience in the outside world, was freeing. And my group mates' stories, whether they mirrored mine or not, gave me validation, or uprooted buried emotions or stunned me into adopting a different perspective on my own situation.

Hearing stories of a person's experience in a conversational context, as in a traditional talk therapy group, told me one thing, but seeing the manner and method by which my group mates' stories were conveyed through visual imagery added multiple layers of meaning. I had entered a singular community of cancer patients and survivors, and my experience of cancer differed from my other group mates' in its details, but I found confirmation of what we shared in the forms of their art.

For example, one panel from Mary E. Walter's comic books shows seven of my group mates sitting around the therapy table, each giving their name and diagnosis. Her asterisk after each name except hers still gives me chills of sadness—it leads to a footnote, "R.I.P." Mary so beautifully memorialized these group members and our loss of them—I don't know how I ever could have expressed that. "Am I Cancer-y Enough," the title of one of her books, also hinted at the feelings I experienced as a cancer survivor who did not have to undergo chemotherapy. In a setting with other cancer patients and survivors whose treatments and prognoses were sometimes a great deal worse than mine, it was a struggle not to compare, to let myself grieve over my own situation without self-consciousness or guilt (Figure 4.1).

Through witnessing and processing with my fellow artists, I was able to transform and externalize that internal experience into something beautiful, even if it expressed an ugliness. From my fear of ovarian cancer and my dark struggle over whether to remove my ovaries came the piece *Living With a Ticking Clock* (2008, acrylic and collage on paper, 19″ × 24″). The therapist first asked us to paint three or four pieces of paper, then asked us to cut them up to create a collage and gave the prompt "create a still life." I painted the three papers silver, red-orange and brown-orange. As a surface for the collage, I created a foreground of silver with a background of deep blue. Two silver ovary flowers with orange fallopian tube stems stick out from the sides of a womb-shaped brown vase sitting on the silver foreground. An ethereal silver bra, shining against the blue background, floats above the vase. The "still life" format of the piece perfectly

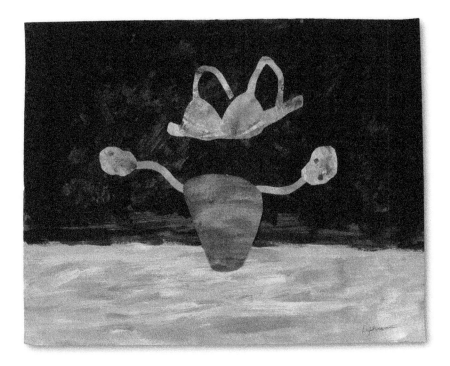

Figure 4.1 Corinne Lightweaver, "Living with a Ticking Clock," 2008, Acrylic Paint.

reflected my dilemma at the time. After being diagnosed with lymphoma and breast cancer, I had learned through genetic testing that I was at high risk for ovarian cancer. The question: Should I cut out working organs to eradicate the specter of a third cancer? The still life expressed the feeling of holding my breath, seemingly forever, as I struggled to find the "right" decision.

Finding witnesses

In art therapy, witnessing happens when you share a room and creative space with people to whom you don't need to explain your predicament or how it has turned your life on its head. This simple gift means everything.

As my life was turned upside down, I had to carry on. My child started kindergarten a few days after my diagnosis. She needed me. One of my wife's biggest fears, when we considered becoming parents, was ending up as a single parent. As she and I faced my second cancer (I had experienced

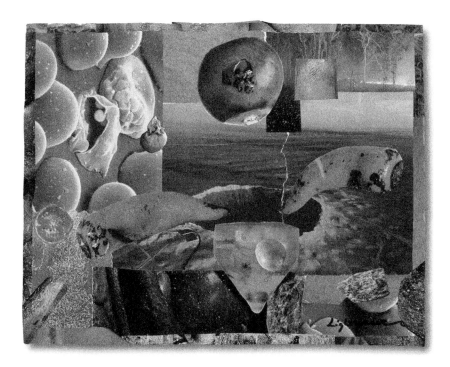

Figure 4.2 Corinne Lightweaver, "Bloodbath," 2009, Collage.

a lymphoma diagnosis four years earlier), we had to hold ourselves together. We had to deal with clinical talk from doctors focused on surgical procedures and nothing else. We had to deal with well-meaning friends, family and strangers whose face and affect toward me changed—sometimes permanently—when they heard the news (Figure 4.2).

In the therapy room, I could share my piece *Bloodbath* (2009, collage on paper, 11″ × 14″) without fear of suddenly sympathetic eyes and tongue clucks, without fear of a veil or even a wall rising up between me and the other person when the word cancer was mentioned. I could remain in my own feelings without feeling the need to reassure the other person that it "wasn't so bad." Without hearing "If there's anything I can do...," the refrain of those outside of cancer who feel helpless and immobilized.

In *Bloodbath*, my fears about my upcoming oophorectomy (removal of the ovaries) coexist with a self-mocking humor. Blackened red peppers, magnified cellular structures, a ghostly pomegranate, snippets of trees on fire and the cavernous opening of a volcano, all combine with other images to create a ghastly, bloody collage that suggests a womb and fallopian tubes. The images reflect my deepest revulsion about surgery on my own body while at the same time overdramatizing the situation in order to make light of it.

Finding the truth in distortion

Autobiographical art is by nature distorted—if it were not, it would be a documentary. As I made art, I did not aim for documentation. Even if I had, I could not have been objective about my own life. As a former journalist, I think about these things. All art, all description, all writing is subjective. And for the most part, that's what's interesting about it.

Creating art in the therapy space allowed me to obtain distance from painful truths or fantasies while still letting them surface. It also allowed me the possibility of delving into fears and admitting them. Experiencing some of my pieces as overdramatic gave me the freedom to laugh at myself or at least take refuge from the pain I experienced; overdramatization also let me dive under the numb exterior to feel suppressed frustrations, anger and sadness.

The seven-month period of wearing expanders—balloons of saline— under the skin in preparation for breast reconstruction was excruciating. Through *Still Life with Knives* (2008, acrylic, paper, leather and trimming on paper, 14″ × 11″), I was able to express the agony of phantom itching and other artificial sensations, along with real pain. In the painting, a moon of pale flesh rises above a brown leather foreground. Three large knives over-lay the moon-breast shape, which is slashed straight across and bleeding. My family was embroiled in a fight with my health insurance company for coverage of the reconstruction surgery. I felt despair. My attempts to adjust to the foreign objects under my skin gave way to fantasies of cutting out the expanders myself (Figure 4.3).

Resistance is futile

In the art therapy group, I had the opportunity to work with many types of materials and media. Some were familiar to me, some not. Some of those familiar materials could be used in new ways. As we dabbled in the different types of media, I resisted collage because I thought it meant "vision boards"—the kinds of saccharine collages I'd seen created with words and images cut from women's magazines. Peace. Harmony. Prosperity. Because of that belief, I didn't consider collage a legitimate or compelling art form.

Entering the medium of collage through the use of fabric, however, al-lowed me to let go of preconceived notions. The textures and colors of the fabric reminded me of paint. Fabric, like paint, allowed for—and even called for—layering. And I noticed that layers and the nubs of the fabric

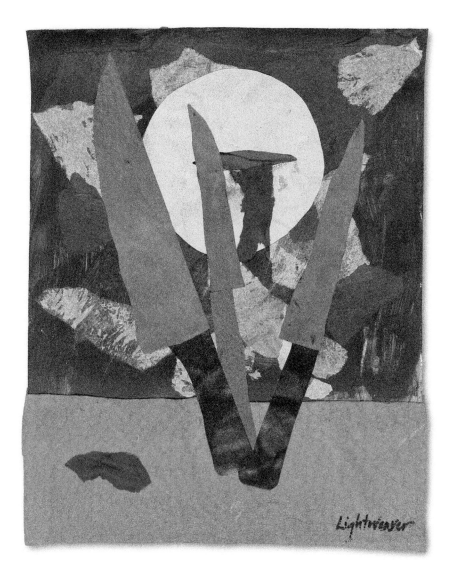

Figure 4.3 Corinne Lightweaver, "Still Life with Knives," 2008, Fabric Collage.

added a texture similar to that which I had achieved in the past with acrylic paint and oils.

When I began creating collages using pictures cut from magazines, the variety of colors, textures and images allowed me to tell a different type of—and sometimes more richly layered—story than those I conveyed with cloth. This medium also engaged my subconscious more, so that only after completing an artwork did I begin to identify, interpret and understand its many messages (Figures 4.4 and 4.5).

My first fabric collage was *Post-Mastectomy Nude with Margarine-Tub Breasts* (2008, 19″ × 14 × 1.5″). Created from cloth and leather pieces glued to paper, the work arose from the therapist's prompt to create a "personal landscape." The image shows a faceless nude, reclining to the left in the style of so many classic paintings. Its creation and my subsequent interpretation of the artwork represented an emotional breakthrough for me. The piece reflects the displacement I felt as I endured the plastic expanders placed under my skin to prepare it for breast reconstruction surgery. The bases of two Styrofoam cups under the brown suede breasts exemplify the distasteful, unnatural, synthetic foreign objects under the skin where my breasts once grew. The two electric-pink leather slashes—vivid scars replacing nipples on the mounds of the breasts—stand in harsh contrast to the soft yellows, beiges and browns in the piece. The scene juxtaposes the harsh technology

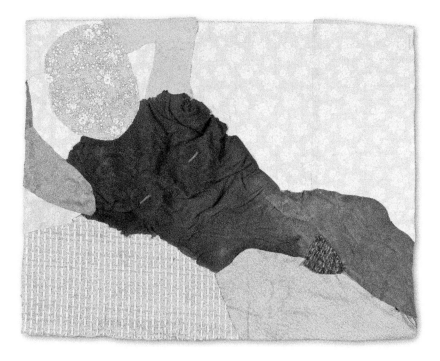

Figure 4.4 Corinne Lightweaver, "Post-Mastectomy Nude with Margarine-Tub Breasts," 2008, Fabric Collage.

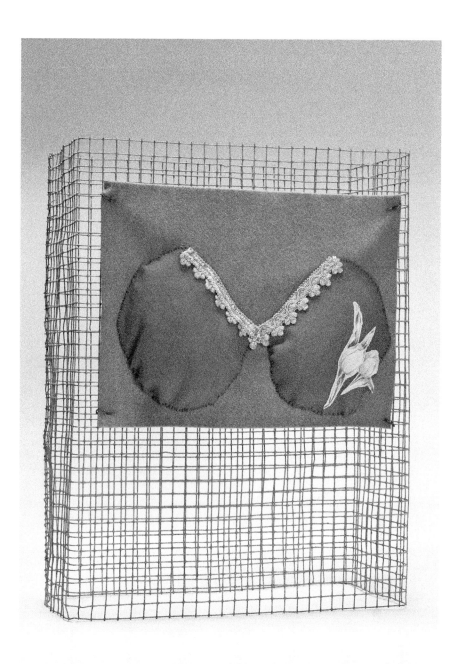

Figure 4.5 Corinne Lightweaver, "Prosthetic Bosom," 2008, Metal Mash and Fabric.

of modern-day surgical techniques with the repose of the classic nude, illustrating my discomfort with the medical intervention in my feminine self-image.

Collage chose me in the creation of that artwork—and resistance was futile. Sometime later, I underwent a similar conversion to assemblage, a three-dimensional version of collage. My first assemblage was *Prosthetic Bosom* (2008, 18″ × 14″ × 7″), created with cloth, cotton, trimming, paper, welded wire mesh and picture hanging wire. As always, the narrative given here came much later, after I created the artwork, which was achieved in a nearly trancelike but also methodical state. This piece examines femininity and motherhood and expresses my feelings of being a living science experiment. A bra—created from red felt, pink trimming, and tulip-patterned cloth decoration—represents an artificial femininity and raises the question of whether femininity, in the absence of breasts, can be restored by *outer* trappings such as clothing. I used blue thread rather than red and hand stitching versus machine sewing because the uneven, visible stitches emphasize that no prosthetic can restore what was originally there. It also draws on Harlow's psychological experiments with baby rhesus monkeys. The red bra is attached to a cold, welded wire framework. In Harlow's experiments, baby monkeys were removed from their biological mothers and confronted with two mannequins, one covered with soft, lifelike fur and the other an uncovered wire armature with an attached "face" and bottle of life-yielding milk. The monkeys always ultimately bonded with the milkless, more tactilely inviting soft mannequin—its softness so powerfully alluring, it compelled them to starve. In this transaction with cancer, as Harlow shows, I lost my bosom, not simply my breasts. My rib cage is represented by the wire framework, no longer supporting actual breasts. I no longer had a bosom to comfort my child or lover. My femininity was in question.

Although at that time I was in the process of breast reconstruction, ultimately this artwork addresses the fact that reconstruction is cosmetic only; it does not treat the interior wounds of the soul, mind and emotions. The use of picture wire to attach the prosthetic bosom I created to the wire frame invokes and underscores the sense of superficial repair.

Prosthetic Bosom affected me deeply. I think that it's not only about what I expressed but what was expressed back to me. My sculpture became my companion; I felt "seen" by my art. Working with tangible materials in hand allowed the intangible feelings in my body and mind to surface.

Give Me Wings (2008, collage on paper, 10″ × 13.5″) was the first piece in which my images extended beyond the border of the artwork. The collage shows a beautiful woman lying under a blanket woven with strings of DNA, gazing upward at a large, big-breasted woman from a Chagall painting floating above her. Wings of blue and green feathers sprout from

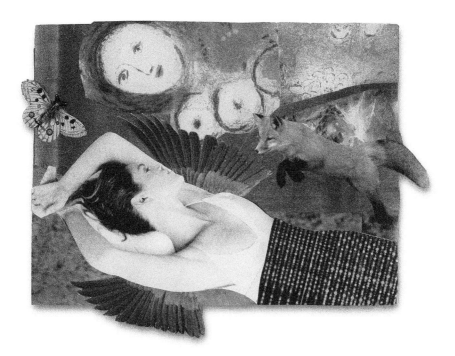

Figure 4.6 Corinne Lightweaver, "Give Me Wings," 2008, Collage.

the prone woman's back. To the left, a butterfly, representing femininity, floats across the edge. To the right, a fox, representing life, leaps from outside the border in. The collage emerged as I awaited surgery to replace the skin expanders under my chest's surface with breast implants. The collage was the only way I could fully express how I longed for deliverance (Figure 4.6).

Developing an internal art therapy space

Just as the patient in traditional therapy may develop the voice of their therapist inside their head—a voice they can draw upon in times of stress—I developed a Traveling Art Therapy Space. The Internal Art Therapist and room full of fellow artists I carried home in my head allowed me to continue to create at home the works that testified to my cancer experience and other life experiences.

At home or elsewhere, I would continue working to the theme of that week or spinning off in my own direction. During the time I participated in the Cancer and Creativity group, some of my most powerful work was

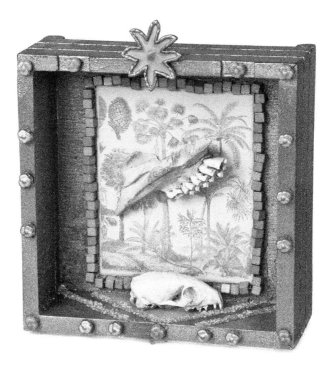

Figure 4.7 Corinne Lightweaver, "Verdant Spring," 2008, Wood Box with Bones.

created or completed at home, including most of my three-dimensional art. But I believe that I could only do so at that time because I transported the space mentally within me. My garage studio became a satellite of the art therapy space (Figure 4.7).

Following the art therapist's prompt of "boxes," I created a number of assemblage pieces at home. *Verdant Spring* (2008, wood, bones, paper, glass, acrylic, 8.25″ × 7.25″ × 3.25″) plays on destruction and rebirth, a recurring theme in my post-cancer work, along with windows. The bottom of a cigar box, painted gold and tipped on its side, creates a framework. Inside, a background of found pale yellow cardboard decorated with spring-green palm trees, bordered by wooden cube-shaped beads, provides the backdrop for a diagonally placed piece of a deer's jaw. A rodent's skull rests in the base of box, surrounded by a triangle of light green beads. Flower-shaped gold and green beads decorate the frame. Some people look at bones as morbid but for me they represent life and the presence of God. In this piece, themes of destruction and rebirth combine in an altar of hope, representing the rebirth that can and did arise, for me, following the destructive force of cancer.

In *Design-A-Tit Kit* (2008, mixed media, 9.75″ × 11″ × 1″), I explore the unfathomable decisions I had to make—often quickly—regarding my breast reconstruction. The options were so unreal to me that I could not fully comprehend and absorb them. The doctor asked me what color and size I wanted my nipples to be. I just wanted to look like myself, like I had always looked. The quaint open-faced wooden storage box in Design-A-Tit Kit belies the horrible decision it references. In the small compartments are buttons, symbolizing nipples, of various shapes, colors and textures. Also included are cardboard spools of thread in four colors. The box is bordered with detailed, feminine, yellow and white trimming. The doctor's question seems like it should be solved with a simple kit or visit to the tailor. Point to the colors and sizes, select the thread, problem solved! Impossible.

Even once the decision was made, the solution was not as simple as the doctor presented. Only when I was lying on the table, as the medical tattooist leaned over me, were the limitations of this cosmetic treatment mentioned. I was told I would have to get the tattoo redone every six months because medical tattoos fade and would fade quicker if I didn't avoid the hot tub and the ocean. However, if I wanted to get retattooed, each time I did so it would further flatten the surgically recreated nipple— so there was no winning. The piece finds humor in such absurdity.

Ribbons befitting a medal of honor grace the top of *Victory Box* (2009, leather, fabric, trimming, wood, acrylic, metal, 3.25″ × 8.25″ × 6.25″), another piece made with a cigar box. I designed the storage box for my sister who, unlike me, chose to use prosthetic nipples rather than have nipple reconstruction surgery. Using leather, fabric, trimming and paint, I created an elegant caselike space for items that can represent pain and loss. *Valiente*, the Spanish word for "brave," appears on the inside lid in the one surface area of the cigar box that is left uncovered. A pillow sewn from blue velvet and gold sparkling fabrics offers a place of honor. Circle imagery on the inside and outside of the box echoes breasts, areolas and the prosthetic nipples. The imagery also elevates the breast and underscores its sacred role in lovemaking and the provision of nourishment.

Making these and other boxes was intensely satisfying. Perhaps creating three-dimensional art is so healing because as a person with cancer, my life was often reduced by doctors and others to a two-dimensional existence. I was not the sum of my life, but the sum of my diagnosis, medical tests and treatment protocols. Three-dimensional art takes up space, as I wished to take up space and be represented in space. Two-dimensional art can be more easily stored and tucked away. Three-dimensional art demands to be seen and takes more care to disguise.

Finding meaning

Cancer can stop art making for some artists. For me, art therapy for cancer brought me back to the creative state and to active art making. The magic of therapeutic art making may not differ much from nontherapeutic art making for some artists. But for me, the dream state of creation under stress and the unconscious revealing of thoughts and emotions occurred at a much deeper level than if I talked or wrote about it. As long as a person who is making art from the unconscious is able to interpret and glean insight, then the setting might not matter. But for me, the therapeutic setting was a necessity for creating transformative, original art that helped me express and come to see the range of emotions my cancer diagnosis and treatment generated.

Chapter 5

Remembering, creating and working through

Loene Trubkin and Esther Dreifuss-Kattan

Artist: Loene Trubkin

I would like to paraphrase Sigmund Freud's 1914 essay "Remembering, Repeating and Working Through" as "Remembering, *Creating* and Working Through." Freud initially saw his method of free association and interpreting dreams as a more active and creative process of remembering that could access the unconscious. Freud, S. (2006). It helped his patients to overcome their resistances to working through psychological issues related to loss and trauma. Some of us may not really remember—or have repressed—our past trauma, while we unconsciously act it out both in the external world in our relationships with others, and within the therapeutic milieu with the psychoanalyst or psychotherapist. Acting out our inner conflicts in an unconscious way is not necessarily to our benefit. A psychotherapeutic relationship allows us to analyze and correct this behavior together with the psychotherapist and to slowly overcome it. Confusing or traumatic early childhood experiences can be retrieved in adult life with the help of the interpretation of dreams, fantasies and particularly through artistic expression, all within the transference of the therapeutic relationship with the therapist or within the dynamic of a therapeutic group setting.

Trauma, derived from the Greek word for "wound," was originally related to a physical injury; Freud understood trauma as an injury to the mind. Cancer traumata affect both the body and mind. A diagnosis of cancer is always a personal encounter with death, followed by shock and acute grief as well as a sense of the disorganization of one's emotions. As mourning one's death initiates a continuing process of remembering, creating and working through is needed to avoid deep and persistent emotional scars. A cancer diagnosis is always experienced by the patient as potentially life-threatening, even though cancer often ends up being a more chronic than acute disease.

Similar to the psychoanalytic processes, the creative, symbolic processes rely heavily on free association and projective techniques to initiate reparation, stabilizing one's sense of self-continuity and thus bringing to the surface unknown and "unthought" feelings (Aragno, 2003). Memories and feelings can be creatively molded and then investigated together within the group of cancer patients who travel very different, even singular cancer journeys, but who also share similar common concerns. What all people with cancer work through in the mourning of their initial trauma is the fear of intrusive, toxic chemotherapies, of multiple surgeries and the loss of a body part or function. A life-threatening illness can highlight earlier repressed psychological wounds, aggravating unresolved individual traumata from early childhood that have not been fully metabolized, such as internal bad objects that were not worked through in the past. Working through the mourning associated with cancer trauma and its related biopsychosocial issues with the help of artistic imagery helps regulate affects such as despair, sadness, and loneliness, resulting in cognitive expansion and the transformation of the self. Some of the helplessness felt is then dispelled (Sollars, 2004). Recollection, reconstruction and restoration open the possibility in the patient for reflection and the transcendence of despair; eventually, even a feeling of gratitude can surface, if real creative psychological reparation does occur (Aragno, 2003).

As we learned from Freud, trauma that is repressed often surfaces gradually through symbolic representation and in the transference relationship with a psychoanalyst. In *Moses and Monotheism*, Freud describes how traumata assume their force by a temporal delay. Initially, patients have no access to the memory, feelings, voices or images of their trauma. While the trauma of a cancer diagnosis with its potential of death is a real event, the overwhelming terror and anxiety that accompany hearing a diagnosis for the first time (in an oncologist's office, perhaps) is often immediately repressed or dislocated, causing the patient to lose emotional access to it. As Cathy Caruth writes: "[trauma] is always the story of a wound that cries out, that addresses us in an attempt to tell us of a reality or truth that is not otherwise available" (Caruth, 1996, p. 4). Repression might be an unconscious survival tactic for the newly diagnosed patient, necessary in order to focus immediately on practical problems like invasive treatment. Despite its utility in the short term, repressing the threat of death and the unknown can lead to numbness and withdrawal from good inner objects, as well from supportive social interactions. Free associations, visualizations, images and creative expressions, as they are interpreted together with the art therapist, can uproot repressed anxiety, keep overwhelming feelings at bay, foster therapeutic transformation and initiate the working through process. These conscious and unconscious memories and experiences are expressed in creative imagery and visualizations but are also acted out within the environment of the therapeutic encounter, with art therapy and psychotherapy reciprocally influencing each other (Leuzinger-Bohleber, 2015).

Trauma is defined today after Freud as a threat of death or of serious injury, compromising both physical and psychological equilibrium, and takes into account the individual's emotional response to these stressful, frightening events. Helplessness, shame, guilt and anger can all be reactions to the stress of exposure (Sharp, Fongay, & Allan, 2012). Cancer can trigger overwhelming anxiety and a feeling of depersonalization, of giving up or being invisible, as the sense of self weakens or even ruptures entirely. One loses basic trust in the functioning of one's world, including medical and family systems of support. In general, traumata are remembered visually, in narrative form, or in fragments; this may become violent or intrusive, as when traumata reappear as nightmares or when sound, smell and color unexpectedly lead back to traumatic memories and provoke retraumatization. Even long after her cancer was cured, a certain ex-patient would taste metal in her mouth whenever she entered a hospital, reliving the side effects of intensive chemotherapy she had undergone many years earlier.

In certain long-term, isolating treatment situations in hospitals, such as bone marrow or stem cell transplantations for blood cancers, patients relate that they experience a total loss of self-agency and harbor strong feelings of neglect in spite of complete medical care. While their medical issues are carefully monitored, their psychological needs are not addressed. Transplantation is a near-death experience, both symbolically and in reality in which the body is brought back from the brink of death through a foreign agent: the patient's own stem cells or bone marrow from a close relative or donor. Perhaps predictably, then, transplantation brings with it a sense of otherness that can cause severe psychological isolation. Once the new cells take hold and the blood counts are slowly balanced, some of this fear recedes, but the vulnerability that comes from physical and psychological trauma can remain for up to a year or two.

Creating art allows a person with cancer to represent and project on canvas or paper what is hidden from consciousness, and thus slowly become aware of their emotional vulnerabilities and their need for support and care. As much as they contemplate their present with a life-threatening illness and anticipate an uncertain future, patients also slowly begin to work with a visual language through their undigested early life. Creativity counteracts powerlessness, doubt, panic and grief; memories as well as experiences from the present become more physically and psychologically integrated, allowing the cancer patient to live more fully in the present.

The strength gained from these pictorial expressions, and from the investigations and interpretations they precipitate, make the person with cancer stronger and more flexible in the face of uncertainty. Talking and associating, patients explore their personal trauma together with the art-psychotherapist. Together with others in their art group, they can "hold" and handle these fears, hopes and experiences that matter so much to them (Caruth, 1995).

Art making searches for the unimaginable. It spurs you to explore somatic and psychic injuries to find a code or language for nonverbal expression. Group participants and their art therapist learn that language in the singular form it takes for each patient-artist; they learn to listen and bear witness to what is expressed from within. This mutual work to comprehend each other is what allows the gratifying solidity of personal narratives to be constructed out of suffering. Imagination alone can address somatic trauma in its psychological effect: combatting a patient's grief and fears of death and mutilation. In the group setting together, however, the more social aspects of trauma may be worked through from all sides: feelings of separateness or togetherness, relations of the self and the other. In dialogue, perhaps ironically, can arise the singular aesthetic form of the personal cancer narrative.

Of course, in such a setting, this dialogue may be one that continues after death. Art can create such a memorial as it is formed in the intersubjective environment of the group. Each member can internalize and reintegrate memories of lost friends into themselves, while remaining aware of how they come to know and display their selves publicly. As a connection to a lost friend is made forever poignant or existing on canvas, it becomes externalized for the self and others through creative work. The artist friend will keep existing in our mind and on the canvas. We do not actually give up or forget the departed friend but rather internalize and reintegrate our memories of her into the self. Creative expression with its potential for integration and mediation is in itself a working through process that allows for externalization, avoiding denial or incomplete mourning. Paintings, collages and sculpture assuage the pain of loss while guiding artist and viewer to reconcile with unsatisfied desires and unfulfilled longing. This potential to fulfill the two tasks of mourning, detachment and continuity, is well demonstrated in Loene Trubkin's artwork and personal narrative in the following section.

Working through

Loene Trubkin

Almost four years after treatment for fallopian tube cancer, I thought I was cured. Why not? Breast cancer diagnosed 32 years earlier had never returned.

I was devastated to learn I was wrong. The gynecological cancer recurred, invading my colon, and requiring a colostomy. This resulted in a nasty postsurgical infection, and ultimately required radiation and brachytherapy, as well as chemotherapy to be put in remission. All the while, I was afraid that those obnoxious treatments heralded the looming end of my life.

A friend then suggested I come to the Healing Arts Group. I could join her there in making art once a week. "But," I said, "I have no talent." She convinced me I would enjoy it anyway and wouldn't be made to feel incompetent. And she was right. Art IS healing, at least as facilitated by Esther Dreifuss-Kattan.

As the weeks went by, working with acrylic paints, fabrics, even colorful masking tape, I found myself freer to try something new, to experiment with abstraction, to let my feelings flow through my imagination. I discovered I love colors, the deeper and more intense the better. I pinned dozens of my pieces on the walls of my home and realized I liked them. I smile when I see them there. They make my rooms brilliant with color and vivid with meaning. Even the sad pieces, the ones that stem from the deaths of compatriots in my cancer support group, remind me of the life force that sustains us through hard times.

The Healing Arts Group is an oasis for my creative self, for the part of me that is not about illness or treatment or fear of the next scan results. For two hours a week, I forget that I am a cancer patient. I express what I feel at that moment. I work through feelings about my family, about the woods and the beach, about color and texture and placement. I decide if lines should be straight or curved, how to make the moon shine through trees, when a project is finished, whether a piece is worth saving. I create the art, and it's mine to exhibit or to trash. In this one area of my life, I am in complete control.

Just before the Healing Arts group meets, I see my psychoanalyst of many years. Issues generated in those sessions find their way into my art. I work through what it's like to see or be seen, to feel free or trapped, to trust or not. I try to imagine what joy looks like, and sorrow. I think about what symbolizes my relationships with people and places. I try to follow Esther's admonition to think less, to let it all go and give my right brain room to run.

Our lives are always in transition, and they are not always smooth and easy transitions. For cancer patients, the thought of transitioning from life to death hovers. Those who find comfort in cancer support groups are frequently reminded of their own mortality by the death of fellow patients. Feeling kicked in the stomach by loss, they simultaneously need to celebrate those lives, the lives that could be their own. Picture 1 is as an effort to work through one death, that of a young, vital mother of two whose life touched mine in weekly support group sessions for three years (Figure 5.1).

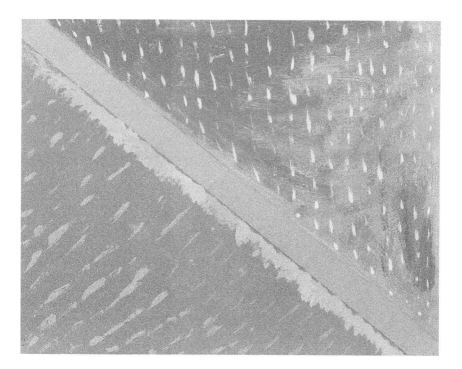

Figure 5.1 Loene Trubkin, "Sally's Grotto," 2013, Acrylic on Paper.

The diagonal blue masking tape pulls life and death, polar opposites, into the same frame while emphasizing their contrasts. On the left, the sparkling blue-green ocean runs up onto the shore, a symbol of light and life. On the right, the gray sand absorbs grieving tears as they fall from a darkened sky (Figure 5.2).

Child rearing is different now, but I grew up in the 1940s and 1950s, when children were expected to be seen and not heard. Parents defined their responsibilities in terms of shelter and nutrition and education, not child development. I grew up believing my thoughts were of interest to no one, even myself, and expressing them proved dangerous. Muzzling or gagging myself became a way to protect myself. Remaining silent became habitual. Even when I wanted to speak, I found it very difficult. Inside was a chorus of voices telling me that disaster awaits any spontaneity. Now that cancer has made my mortality more real to me, I want to speak about my life and yet I find that words are still too dangerous. Art provides another avenue, one in which I can express my feelings and not feel endangered (Figure 5.3).

See salmon swimming upstream, leaping waterfalls to reach their destination, their spawning grounds. They don't eat, they don't rest and they

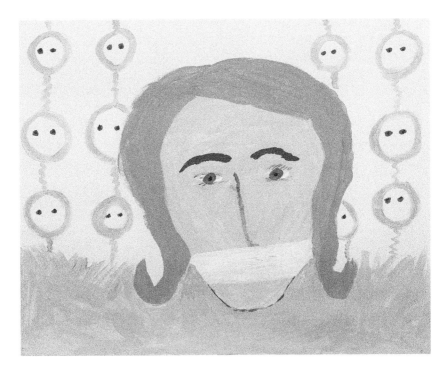

Figure 5.2 Loene Trubkin, "Gag Order," 2013, Acrylic on Paper.

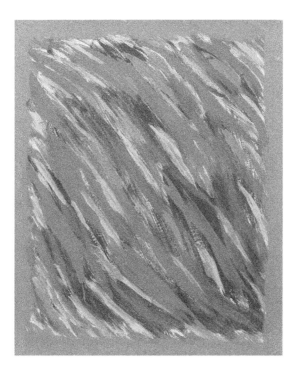

Figure 5.3 Loene Trubkin, "Change," 2014, Acrylic on Paper.

ignore injuries and predators seeking their flesh. They remind me of cancer patients, also swimming upstream against the current, fighting to survive. Sometimes they forget why it's so important to stay alive. Is it to be here when a cure is discovered? Or to see a daughter marry or a grandson graduate? Or simply because life calls to us just as it calls to the salmon? There are days when the sun shines, and dolphins swim along the shore and light and color bring joy to our hearts. How could we leave voluntarily and not wring every bit of joy from our lives? And if that joy disappears on other days because of nausea and mouth sores and radiation burns and all the other horrible side effects, will the joy we do experience be any less vibrant or desired? (Figure 5.4).

My psychotherapist taught me self-hypnosis and encouraged me to create a special place in my mind, a place of security and peace and unconditional love. The place I chose reflects a childhood among the hills and pines of northern California. My mountains and grassy dells, trees, flowers, bees and birds, streams and shrubs, flourish in the sunshine and a lovely cool breeze. I run there with my dog, a clone of the dachshund that soothed my teen years, and I lie in the grass and admire purple mountain majesties. Once again I become calm enough to allow another scan, another infusion,

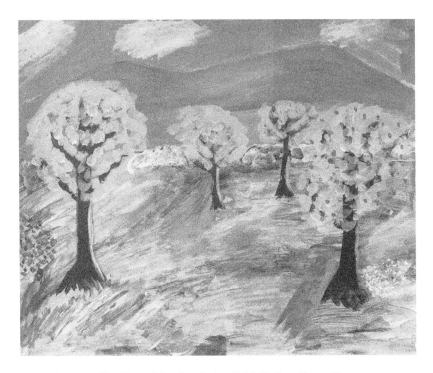

Figure 5.4 Loene Trubkin, "No Confusion," 2017, Acrylic on Paper.

another surgery, another invasion of my body. I can enjoy the flora and fauna thriving in my special place while the doctors' tools shut down cancer cells' growth paths.

Together with me, the art therapist, patients like Loene embark on a creative cancer journey, documenting the fluctuating emotional states of different cancer treatments, reoccurring tests and fruitful or frustrating dialogues with oncologists, as well as with health professionals, family and themselves. We visually share the gains and losses that come with a diagnosis of cancer, engendering trust and hope. Cancer is in many ways defined by loss: you can lose multiple body parts or functions, or an entire body; there is the loss of a career, a job; the loss of friends who are left behind along the way because they could not empathize with cancer stories, and the absent friends who were members of the "Cancer and Creativity" and "Healing Arts" support groups. The gain, on the other hand, begins in the intimacy of these same groups, which exist to share memories and feelings through art, and to stay together through every pitch of the rollercoaster. The group members come to a deep self-knowledge, the yield of frightening truths found in their voyages into the unconscious. Expressing the multiple issues related to cancer, family and the world we live in, the artists' extraordinary perspective can even lead them to joy, balanced on a narrow perch between illness and health.

References

Aragno, A. (2003). Transforming Mourning: A New Psychoanalytic Perspective on the Bereavement Process. *Psychoanalysis and Contemporary Thought, 26* (4), 427–462.

Caruth, C. (1995). *Trauma: Explorations in Memory*. Baltimore, MD: Johns Hopkins University Press.

Caruth, C. (1996). *Unclaimed Experience*. Baltimore, MD: Johns Hopkins University Press.

Freud, S. (1937–1939). Moses and Monotheism. In A. Richards (Ed.), *The Standard Edition of the Complete Psychological Works of Sigmund Freud: Moses and Monotheism: An Outline of Psychoanalysis and Other Works* (Vol. 23) (J. Strachey, Trans.) (pp. 7–137). London: Hogarth Press and the Institute of Psychoanalysis.

Freud, S. (2006). Remembering, Repeating and Working Through. In A. Phillips (Ed.), *The Penguin Freud Reader* (pp. 391–401). London: Penguin Books.

Leuzinger-Bohleber, M. (2015). *Finding the Body in the Mind: Embodied Memories, Trauma, and Depression*. London: Karnac Books.

Sharp, C., Fongay, P., & Allan, J.G. (2012). Posttraumatic Stress Disorder: A Social-Cognitive Perspective. *Clinical Psychology: Science and Practice, 19* (3), 229–240.

Sollar, F.R. (2004). Mourning, Trauma, and Working Through. *Psychoanalytic Review, 91* (2), 201–219.

Winnicott, D.W. (1971). *The Maturational Process and the Facilitating Environment*. New York: International University Press.

Winnicott, D.W. (1974). *Playing and Reality*. New York: Basic Book, Inc.

Chapter 6

Art as lifesaver
Photography, Facebook and installation

Devon Raymond and Esther Dreifuss-Kattan

Artist: Zizi Raymond

Devon Raymond

When I heard a fellow caregiver in a friends and family support group say one night, "My mother is dying of cancer," I realized I had something to offer. Since her mother's diagnosis was new, full of uncertainty, which could also mean full of hope, I told her that perhaps she could look at it the way I had lately come to see my sister's situation. Zizi wasn't dying of cancer. She was living with cancer. It wasn't that Zizi's circumstances were less serious than that of the young woman's mother. It was that Zizi's focus was on living, not dying. To be fair though, she'd had a lot of practice. She'd been living with breast cancer for nearly 20 years.

Zizi was first diagnosed in 1994 when she was just 33 years old. Her oncologist at the time said her prognosis was good because the cancer was not found in the lymph nodes harvested beneath her arm during a lumpectomy. But many months after chemotherapy and radiation, Zizi found a new growth at her breastbone. In a rare occurrence, the cancer had migrated to the lymph nodes beneath her sternum. After undergoing another surgery, which involved removing part of the bone, she received a stem cell transplant at the City of Hope hospital to ensure that any microscopic cancer cells were destroyed.

For nearly ten years, she was deemed to be cancer free. Then in 2005, in another rare occurrence, a new cancer with a different pathology developed in her other breast. This time, it hadn't been caught early. But Zizi still managed to keep it at bay until 2008 when yet another diagnosis would change her life dramatically. The cancer had spread to her liver, adrenal glands and brain.

All of the oncologists she saw in the first week of re-diagnosis agreed that her brain was the priority. She was "lucky," some of them said, because most breast cancers in the brain were small lesions scattered throughout, whereas hers appeared to be a single mass that could be resected with surgery. When Zizi and I met with Dr. Black, the renowned brain surgeon at Cedars Sinai in Los Angeles, we hoped he would calm the anxiety produced by what seemed like a catastrophic diagnosis. But Dr. Black was a reserved man, seeming to save his energy for the operating room. Instead of offering information, he waited for our questions. Zizi, always interested in the body and how it works, asked how he would do the surgery. We had already gathered some information about surgeons who "opened and closed" vs. those who did only the delicate task of removing the tumor. Dr. Black would not open Zizi's skull, nor would he close it. He would, he said, "tease out the tumor" from the complex web of her brain. The word "tease" hung in the air with the gravity of the impending invasion of her brain. We waited through more silence before Dr. Black spoke about the complications that could arise from the surgery. Because of where the tumor was located, Zizi's language and eyesight might be affected. Zizi came to attention. "I don't care about words," she said, "But I need my eyes. I'm an artist."

I was never sure if there really was a choice between Zizi's language and her sight, but she came through the surgery with her vision intact, losing only some peripheral vision. She lost many words. She also lost dates, math and time. And though she regained a good deal of her language, time seemed to be a concept that was lost forever. It wasn't a problem she dwelled on. She had her eyes.

Zizi continued to improve, but the new deficits in her cognitive abilities made her unable to return to her teaching job at the Art Institute of California in Santa Monica. Though this was a major alteration in her life, she also saw it as an opportunity to spend more time on her own art. But her brain had shifted. She didn't know if she was still the same artist. If she couldn't track time, could she still tap into the source from which she produced a large body of work shown and sold in galleries throughout her lengthy career?

Zizi's earliest works consisted mainly of large-scale sculptures made with found objects. She later turned to collages and drawings on canvas, which depicted cutout figures connected to domestic objects with taut lines. The figures strain to maintain the interdependent lines in order to keep from undergoing some catastrophe or other. But just before her re-diagnosis, Zizi had moved into a different phase of her work. In her newest drawings, as she wrote in her last artist statement, "…the precarious balance has been replaced by falling. There is no longer tension in the act of preventing the fall. The fall is embraced, and nurtured as an act of ultimate transformation."

Zizi's re-entry into her art after brain surgery came when, through one of her cancer support groups, she learned of the art therapy classes facilitated by Esther. Esther's knowledge and appreciation of art was stimulating to Zizi, and her plans to curate shows for the participants was an opportunity for Zizi to return to a sense of normalcy by preparing her art for public viewing. As the group allowed Zizi to explore her work from her new reality without judgment, Zizi's confidence returned. And though her work changed again, moving into the abstract, she embraced her "fall," as her body and her art underwent a dramatic transformation.

Throughout her participation in art therapy, she continued to receive treatment for her spreading cancer, including harsh chemotherapies, three more surgeries and various forms of brain radiation. She had a fierce will to live, and her oncologist understood that despite the cancer, her 48-year-old body was strong. But in 2010, two years after brain surgery, she underwent her most invasive and dramatic surgery yet. Called a Whipple procedure after the doctor who first performed the surgery, it includes removing the head of the pancreas, the gallbladder, part of the duodenum—which is the uppermost segment of the small intestine—a small portion of the stomach called the pylorus and the lymph nodes near the head of the pancreas. The surgeon then reconnects the remaining pancreas and digestive organs so that the stomach contents flow into the small intestine. Zizi underwent the surgery on the heels of whole brain radiation, which had compromised the part of her brain that stimulates hunger. So in the four months after the Whipple procedure, with an already diminished appetite and food becoming difficult to process from the re-routing of her digestive track, Zizi dropped from 130 pounds to 100 pounds. At 5′ 7″, this was a dangerous weight.

Her oncologist prescribed Marinol, a synthetic THC that came with dizzying side effects and didn't help her eat. As her primary caregiver, I continually brought her a variety of food that I thought would encourage her appetite and be easy to digest. Local friends took her out for meals, and long-distance friends arranged meal programs for delivery. But inevitably, food would stack in Zizi's refrigerator uneaten. In the evenings, I would clear out the spoiled remnants, then sit by her bed with some new meal I thought would be promising, until she waved it off after one bite. When my gentle but persistent encouragement failed, I made flat-out threats of a feeding tube if she didn't eat, but even that didn't produce results. After Zizi fainted one day in the art therapy group, Esther referred her to a nutritionist, who suggested an eating coach. The coach provided menus for simple, high-fat meals and also went to Zizi's house to demonstrate the making of a protein smoothie. For a time, the smoothie seemed to be the only sure thing Zizi could eat, but it wasn't enough for her to gain weight. We were at a critical juncture. Knowing that only she could control what she put in her mouth and swallowed, I sat by her bed one night, staring at the uneaten small cuts of chicken I had prepared for her, and cried.

Zizi would later tell me that it was then that she understood how serious her condition was and decided that she needed to make her eating public in order to be accountable for it. In May of 2011, she started posting photographs to Facebook of the remainder of all of her meals to show what she had, and more importantly, had not eaten. It was a beautiful twist to the standard photos many people share of plates brimming with perfect, bountiful meals on the verge of being devoured. Zizi's photographs were instead a real and raw admission of what she was unable to eat.

Over an eight-month period, the plates in Zizi's photographs gradually showed less remaining food. The empty plates were a sign that she was making progress. Friends commented with encouragement when she shared her steady weight gain numbers along with the photos. Food, Zizi said, was her primary job during that time. And though eating was work, her photography, which she had once used in some of her early collages, became a new creative outlet. The food images were not mere documentation, but deliberate, visually arresting, clean works in color. They satisfied her passion for making art while serving as a means to literally feed her.

When Esther was planning another show for the art therapy participants in 2013, she suggested that Zizi work with her food photographs to create an installation. The work shown here is made up of the photographs in small scale, inserted into jars that signify each month that Zizi accounted for her eating. She dedicated the work to our grandmother, Theresa Riley Grover, who died of pancreatic cancer in 1972.

Esther Dreifuss-Kattan

We met Zizi and some of her sculpture and her fabric mural *Blood Production* in Chapter 2. You read how Zizi needed more surgery that resulted in a lack of hunger and difficulty eating. One day in the group Zizi fainted and as our studio was part of a large oncology office, a nurse came running and then the doctor. She recovered her consciousness relatively fast but we all were in shock. It seemed obvious that Zizi could not drink and eat enough and, as her sister Devon described, that ultimately led to the food coach and to her taking pictures of the leftovers on her plate that she then posted on Facebook for family and friends to cheer her on.

When we were ready to organize the art exhibition at the New Center for Psychoanalysis in Los Angeles entitled "Cancer on the Couch," Zizi wondered what she could exhibit. I mentioned her amazing photography that she had posted online and thought maybe she could create something that would show the viewer that through her artistry and perseverance she had started to eat again. I did not have any idea what Zizi was planning to showcase but had confidence in her great artistic talent and skills. Having known this artist for about four years by that time and observed her abilities, whatever it was, it would be perfect, creative and moving. In spite of metastasized breast cancer, weight loss and impaired peripheral vision, Zizi was a perfectionist and true artist. We had met the week before because Zizi wanted to see the room for the exhibition and we had chosen the specific glass shelves that would showcase her installation.

However, when Zizi arrived to install her project together with Mary, another group member who became close friends with her and who you will meet in Chapter 8, I was amazed. Out of the beautiful bigger photographs with the leftover food pieces, Zizi created very small images of these plates and glued them on a stable but thin background, resulting in hundreds of little half-eaten food plates. In addition, Zizi bought online huge clear glass food containers with round white tops to close them. Then Zizi laid the containers down on the glass shelves and arranged the very small food photograph plates with food images in such a way that they were flowing out of the containers onto the shelves. I suggested she hang the enlarged photos of the same half-eaten plates on the wall behind for the viewer to actually see them in their arresting beauty (Figures 6.1–6.5).

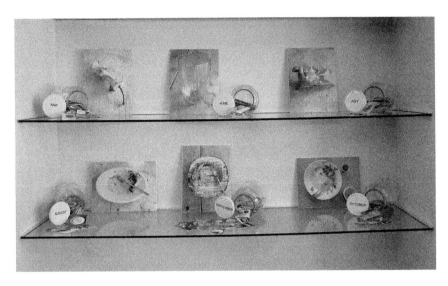

Figure 6.1 Zizi Raymond, "Untitled Installation," 2013.

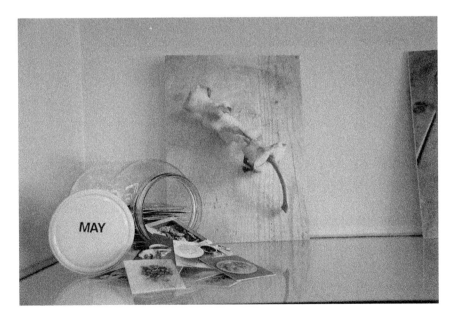

Figure 6.2 Zizi Raymond, detail from "Untitled Installation," 2013.

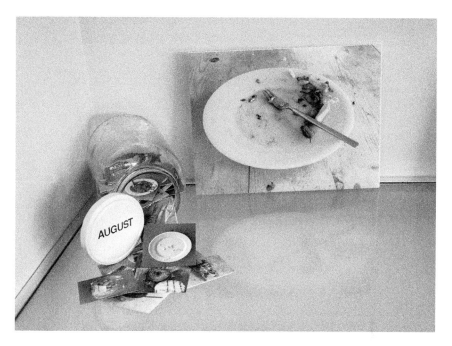

Figure 6.3 Zizi Raymond, detail from "Untitled Installation," 2013.

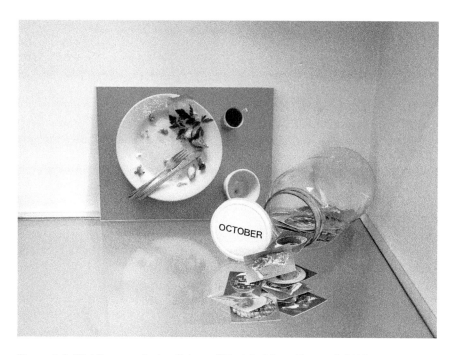

Figure 6.4 Zizi Raymond, detail from "Untitled Installation," 2013.

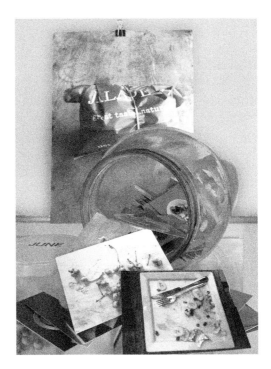

Figure 6.5 Zizi Raymond, detail from "Untitled Installation," 2013.

JARS

Jar 1 *May*, Zizi Raymond, 2013, Photographs and glass jar, 10″ × 6″ × 6″.
Jar 2 *June*, Zizi Raymond, 2013, Photographs and glass jar, 10″ × 6″ × 6″.
Jar 3 *July*, Zizi Raymond, 2013, Photographs and glass jar, 10″ × 6″ × 6″.
Jar 4 *August*, Zizi Raymond, 2013, Photographs and glass jar, 10″ × 6″ × 6″.
Jar 5 *September*, Zizi Raymond, 2013, Photographs and glass jar, 10″ × 6″ × 6″.
Jar 6 *October*, Zizi Raymond, 2013, Photographs and glass jar, 10″ × 6″ × 6″.
Jar 7 *November*, Zizi Raymond, 2013, Photographs and glass jar, 10″ × 6″ × 6″.
Jar 8 *December*, Zizi Raymond, 2013, Photographs and glass jar, 10″ × 6″ × 6″.

Hearing me describing this installation process together with Zizi and Mary may sound very straightforward, as we all know how to arrange and hang up art on our walls at home or put an art object on a nice stand. However, there was nothing easy or straightforward in arranging this particular installation. Mary had picked Zizi up in her car, as she was not allowed to drive any longer due to her vision. She was unfortunately already very thin and pretty weak, as her cancer had progressed significantly. I was stunned to see that Zizi was able to create these amazing little food images so precisely with an X-Acto knife, each the same size, and had glued them to another background so that they looked flat and stable. I could not fathom how Zizi had the patience to search for the perfect jars on her computer and actually had first ordered other ones that she had to send back, as they did not please her aesthetic taste. To stage this installation with different explanation tags next to each jar and describing the month they represented, to have the food flowing out of these jars just to look perfectly natural and to place the bigger photo images, just the right way behind the jars on the wall between the glass shelves, amounted to an amazing focus, concentration and stamina from our very weak artist friend. Every 15 minutes I ordered the three of us to sit down and rest, and I brought water to drink, as I was worried that this entire idea was just not really manageable for Zizi. I was afraid that I had overestimated her strength and that I should not have encouraged this entire project.

However, I also observed, in spite of acute and overwhelming exhaustion, how excited Zizi was, how she conducted herself in a laser-focused professional way and how wonderfully empathic and helpful Mary was to Zizi in the same professional, warm and kind way. It became clear to me that installing this beautiful art piece that the artist had contemplated and had created over many months in her home studio in a precise, professional and highly creative manner was one of the reasons that had kept this artist alive. As the cheering of her friends on Facebook encouraged her to keep eating more with the help of the photographs of her half empty plates, so creating, preparing for and mounting the art installation helped Zizi focus her attention in the present on her artistic work. It illustrated her unconscious attempt to hold on to a future and to life itself, keeping at bay the real threat of death. Art making allowed Zizi to keep working as an artist as she did throughout her adult life, on a smaller and different scale, but with the same focus and talent as her physical state allowed. She was thus able to arrest time. It was less the unconscious process with its psychological message that Zizi was interested in, but rather all her art pieces as you will have read earlier, focused on the new and changing reality of her daily life with cancer and the new symptoms she needed to work through creatively. As the artist used the symbol of circular compositions, representing her blood cells or cancer cells in varied art material earlier in the group, or worked with clay and plastic forks or old slides from medical books or with her favorite Caran D'Ache water soluble crayons, creative activity kept her active and in charge of her life and her art.

Focusing on art making and installing it helped Zizi in coping with the fast progression of her cancer and its trauma, counteracting physical and psychic pain, with its helplessness and fear of dependency and loss. Expressing and creating art meant positive progress and spelled out a sort of recovery and a working through process. It marked a creative response to her ongoing traumatic situation. Creativity and artistic focus counteracted the patient's helplessness and the loss of some physical abilities such as driving and aided in the artistic expansion of her self, forming a bond with good internal objects and a sense of inner connection that allowed for meaningful and emotional relations with others in the group. Expression through art made it possible for Zizi to experience the continuity of life and was also a panacea against pain and physical weakness by fostering the integration of the self. It helped her in adapting to the progression of her cancer with its devastating metastatic way of life. Creating focused Zizi and made mourning tolerable, while repressing it in her daily life. This immensely creative and talented cancer patient had to focus and invite creative activity into her life again to augment effects of joy and pride, helping her by staying away from self-pity, sadness, multiple losses and extreme personal vulnerability.

Creative transformation through art and a close bond to her psychotherapist helped this traumatized artist—who battled breast cancer for 20 years and who was confronted with a traumatic object loss—to regain a coping strategy. As she seemed to repress conscious knowledge of her symptoms and her approaching death, she regained self-agency, counteracting regression and fragmentation in order to contain the panic of mortality. Art making transformed her unconscious world, her self and her internal object representations. She mentioned more often the close relationship she used to have to her grandmother that she missed. Being actively creative in this end stage of life changed Zizi's thinking and feeling in the present. Expression through art and the close object relationship for four years with me, the group art-psychotherapist, provided some relief of physical and psychological symptoms and augmented her appreciation of herself as a creative person. It also secured for her an even closer attachment to her sister Devon and the rest of her loving family, as well as to her friend Mary, to other group members and to her many friends in the greater Los Angeles artistic community.

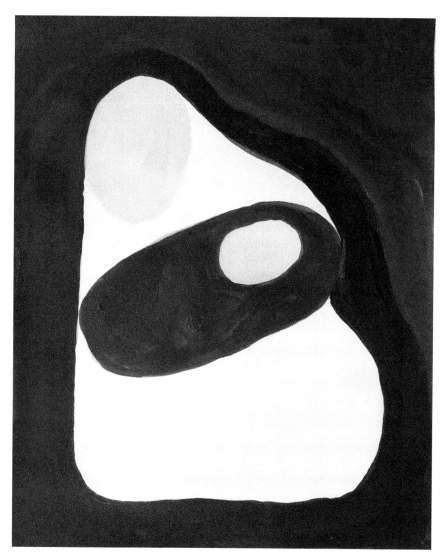

Figure 1.1 Teresa O'Rourke, "Mother and Infant," 2018, Acrylic Paint.

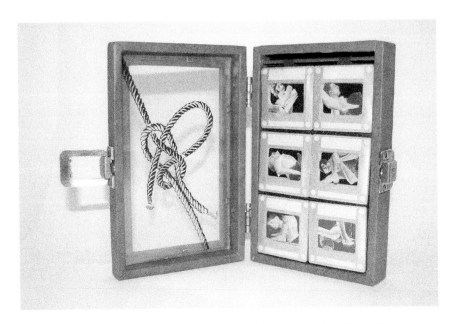

Figure 2.1 Zizi Raymond, "Untitled," 2010, Wood Box with Glass Window and Slides.

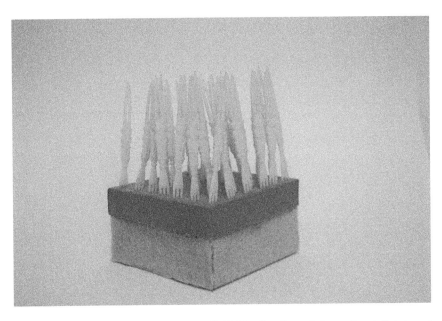

Figure 2.3 Zizi Raymond, "Fork Box," 2008, Cardboard Box, Acryl Paint and Plastic Forks.

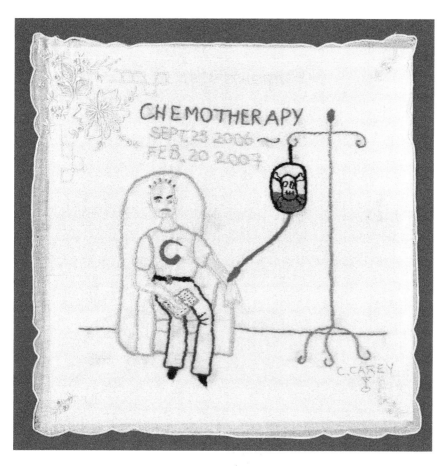

Figure 3.1 Christine Carey, "Chemotherapy," 2012, Embroidery on Vintage Handkerchief.

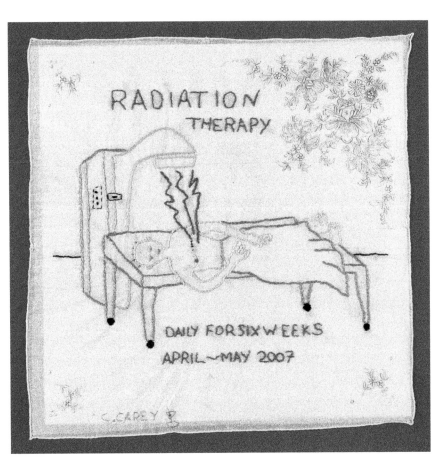

Figure 3.2 Christine Carey, "Radiation Therapy," 2012, Embroidery on Vintage Handkerchief.

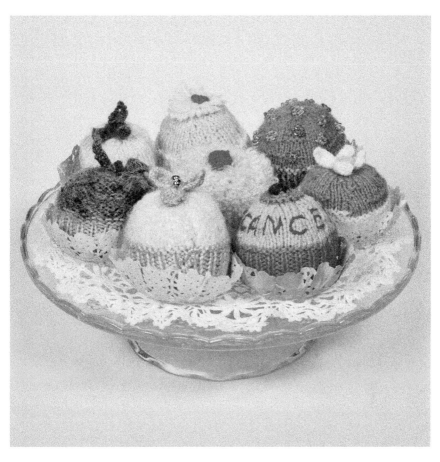

Figure 3.4 Christine Carey, "Mastectomy," 2012, Embroidery on Vintage Handkerchief.

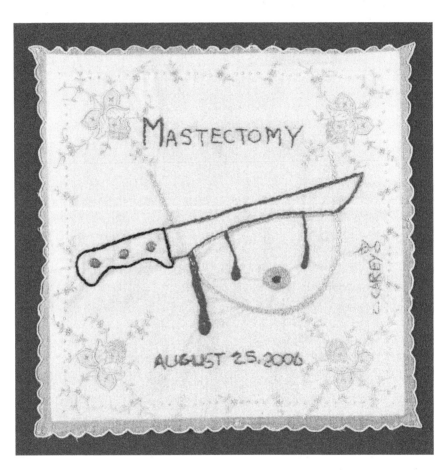

Figure 3.5 Christine Carey, "One in Eight," 2012, Knitting Wool and Paper.

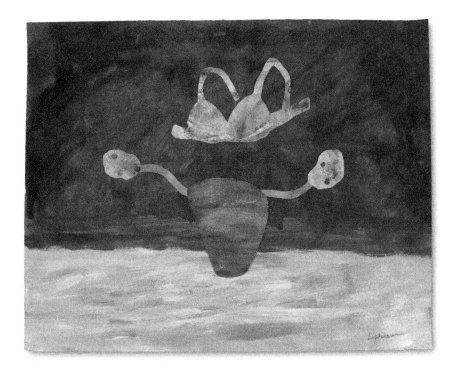

Figure 4.1 Corinne Lightweaver, "Living with a Ticking Clock," 2008, Acrylic Paint.

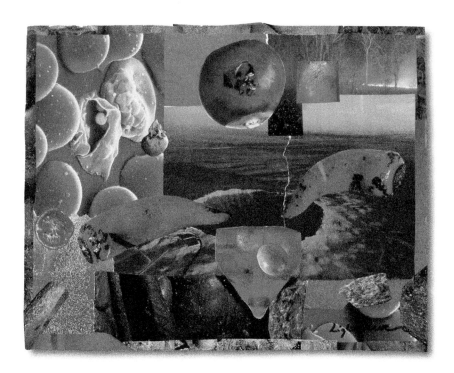

Figure 4.2 Corinne Lightweaver, "Bloodbath," 2009, Collage.

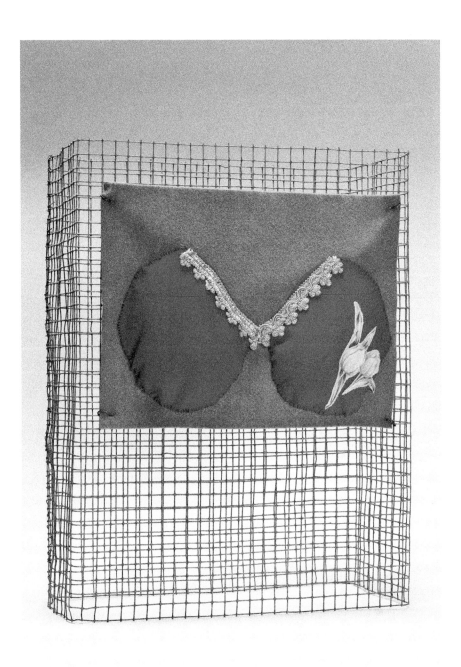

Figure 4.5 Corinne Lightweaver, "Prosthetic Bosom," 2008, Metal Mash and Fabric.

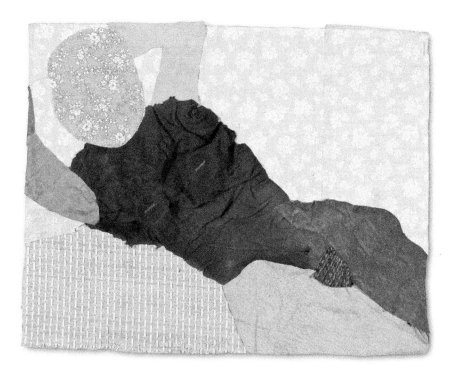

Figure 4.4 Corinne Lightweaver, "Post-Mastectomy Nude with Margarine-Tub Breasts," 2008, Fabric Collage.

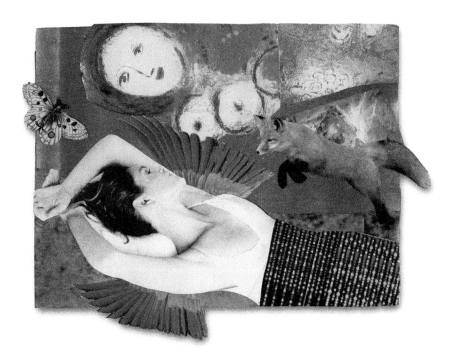

Figure 4.6 Corinne Lightweaver, "Give Me Wings," 2008, Collage.

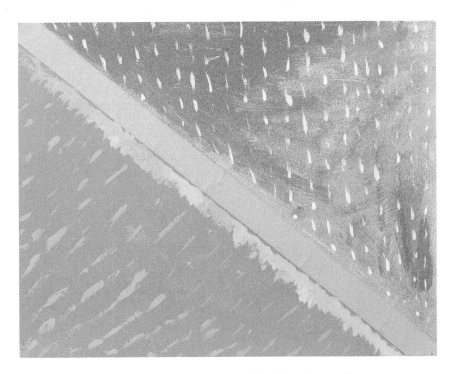

Figure 5.1 Loene Trubkin, "Sally's Grotto," 2013, Acrylic on Paper.

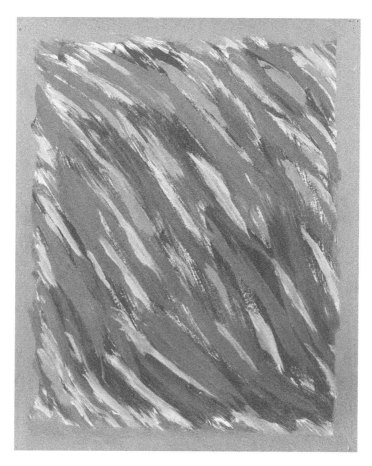

Figure 5.3 Loene Trubkin, "Change," 2014, Acrylic on Paper.

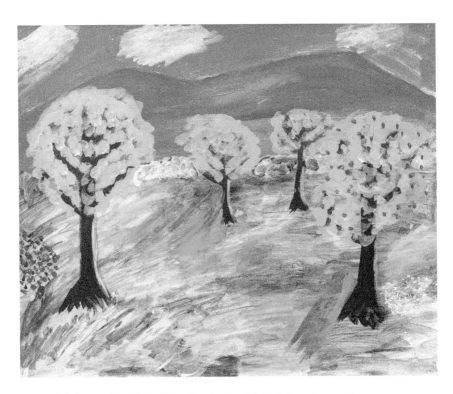

Figure 5.4 Loene Trubkin, "No Confusion," 2017, Acrylic on Paper.

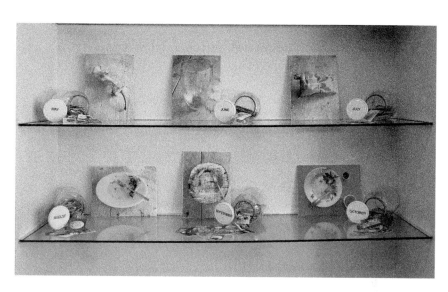

Figure 6.1 Zizi Raymond, "Untitled Installation," 2013.

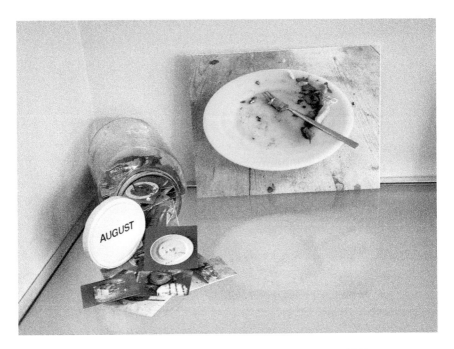

Figure 6.2 Zizi Raymond, detail from "Untitled Installation," 2013.

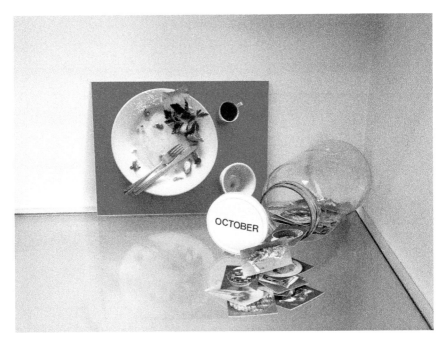

Figure 6.3 Zizi Raymond, detail from "Untitled Installation," 2013.

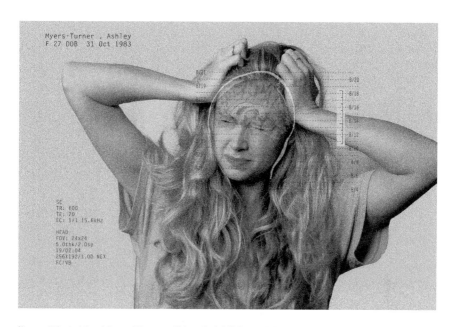

Figure 7.1 Ashley Myers-Turner, "Untitled 1," Digital Photography and MRI, 2011.

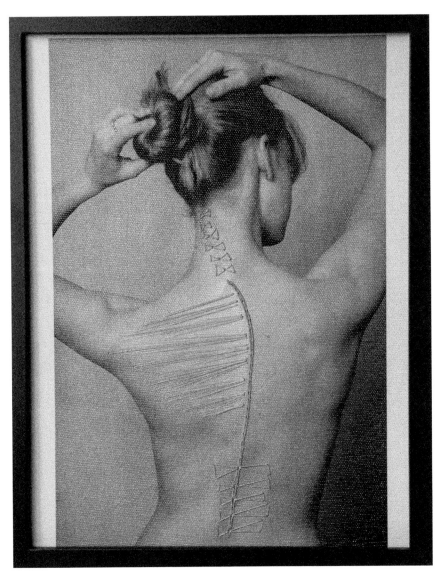

Figure 7.2 Ashley Myers-Turner, "Spine," Digital Photography and Embroidery, 2012 Embroidery.

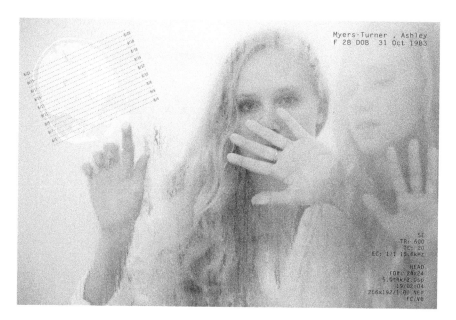

Figure 7.3 Ashley Myers-Turner, "Untitled 2," Digital Photography and MRI, 2011.

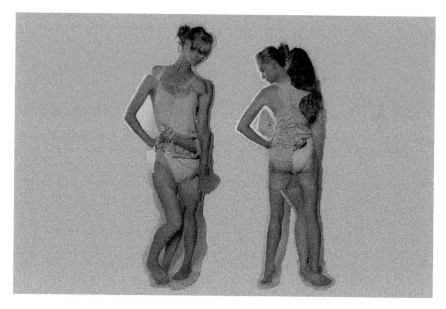

Figure 7.4 Ashley Myers-Turner, "Ashley in Wonderland," Digital Collage, 2011.

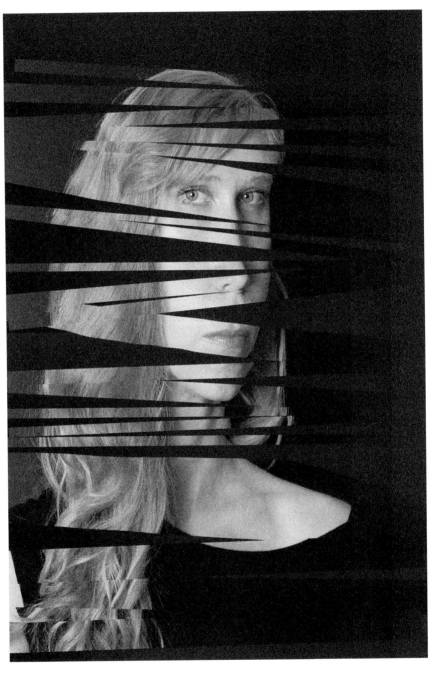

Figure 7.5 Ashley Myers-Turner, "Split Head I," Digital Photography, 2011.

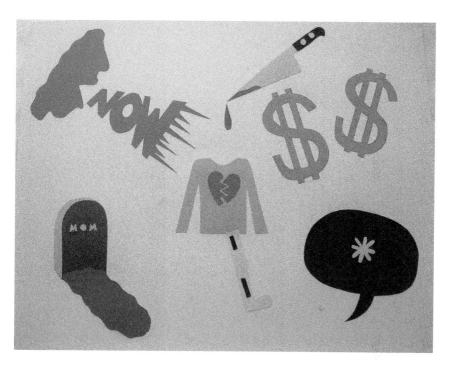

Figure 8.1 Mary E. Walter: "My Immediate Family," color construction paper on Bristol paper, 2009.

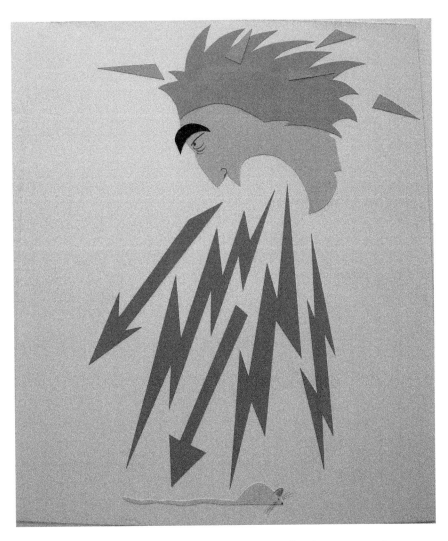

Figure 8.2 Mary E. Walter: "Please Call Me Doctor," color construction paper, graphite pencil on Bristol paper, 2010.

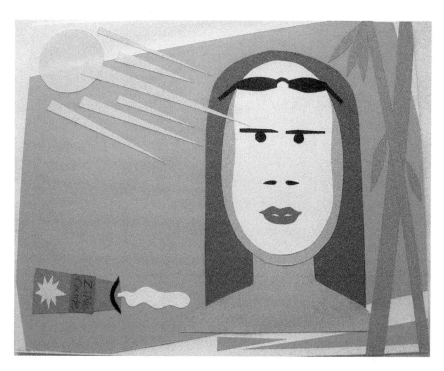

Figure 8.4 Mary E. Walter: "Kabuki? Noh? Sunscreen Mask," color construction paper, Felt Marker on Bristol, 2010.

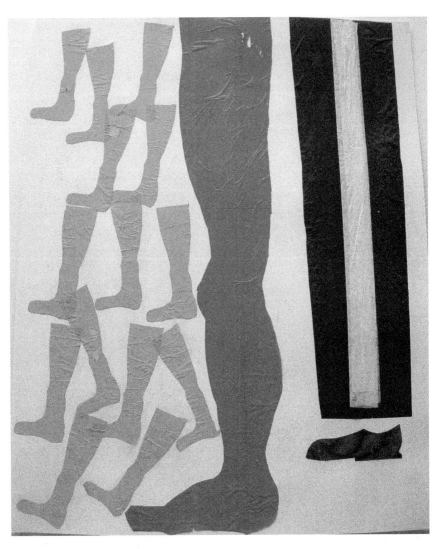

Figure 8.5 Mary E. Walter: "Last Day of Art Therapy: Tissue Paper," fabric on Bristol paper, 2012.

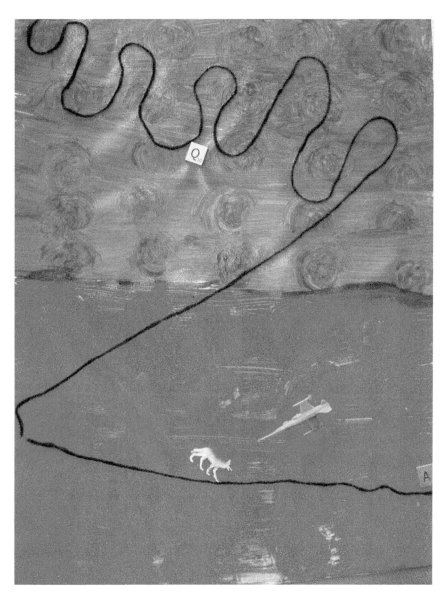

Figure 9.1 Jeff, "My Cancer Map," Acrylic, Plastic Fire, Wool, Scrabble Piece, 2013.

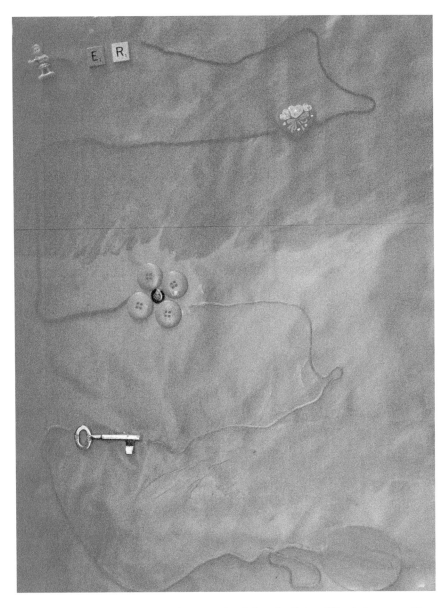

Figure 9.2 Chaya Spatler, "My Cancer Map," Acrylic Paint, Wool, Buttons, Plastic Plate, Metal Key.

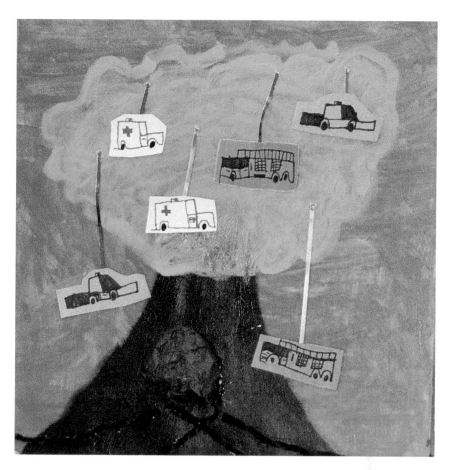

Figure 9.3 Adam Pomeranz, "Tree of Life-My Rescue Tree," Acrylic Paint, Paper, Magic Marker.

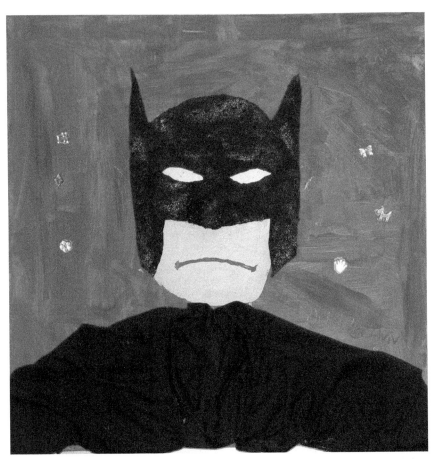

Figure 9.5 Ari, "Self-Portrait-Superhero: Batman," Acrylic Paint, Lack Felt, Glass Beads.

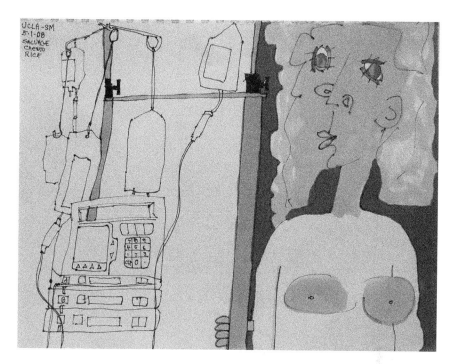

Figure 10.1 Howard Bass, "Salvage Chemo Ride," 2008.

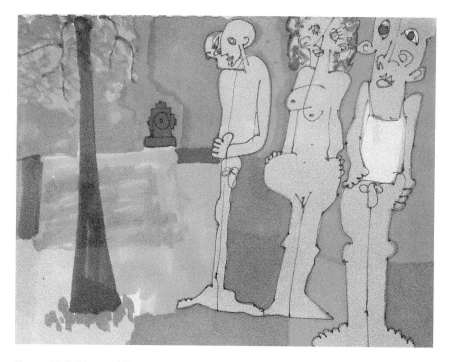

Figure 10.2 Howard Bass, "Untitled," 2008.

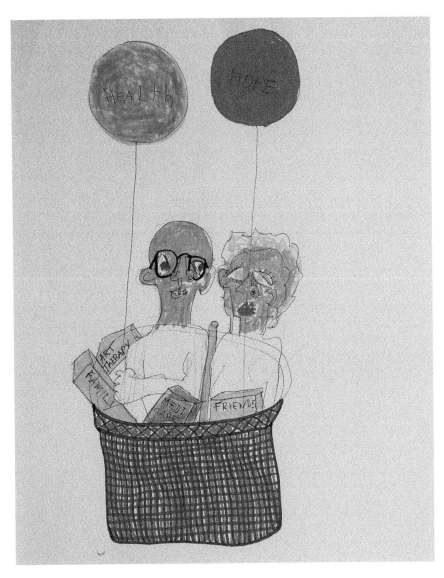

Figure 10.4 Howard Bass, "Basket of Blessings," 2009.

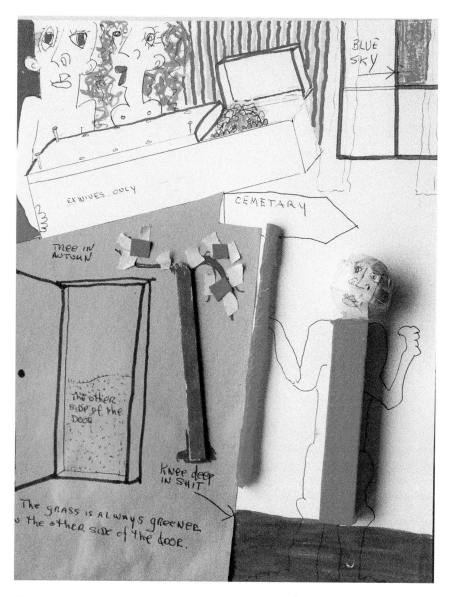

Figure 10.5 Howard Bass, "Knee Deep in Shit," 2009.

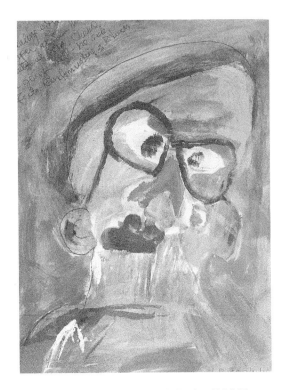

Figure 10.6 Howard Bass, "Two Portraits: A Dialog," 2009.

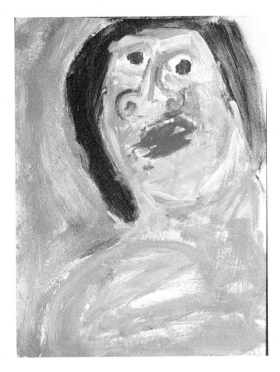

Figure 10.7 Howard Bass, "Two Portraits: A Dialog," 2009.

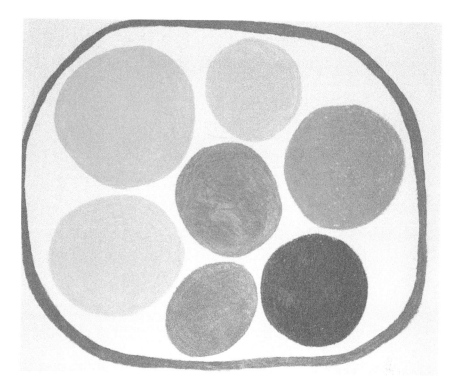

Figure 10.8 Zizi Raymond: "Circles," Acrylic Paint.

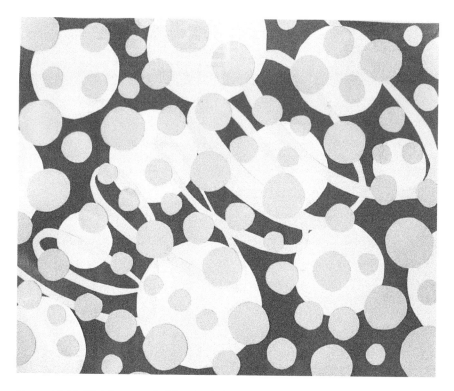

Figure 10.10 Zizi Raymond: "Circles," Acrylic Paint.

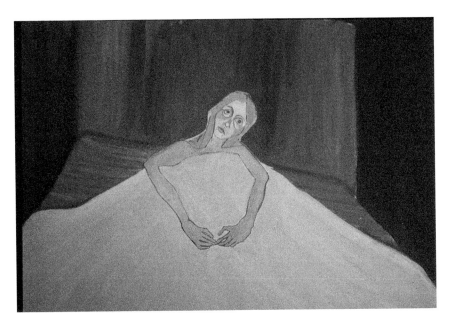

Figure 10.13 Esther Dreifuss-Kattan: "Distance," Acrylic Paint on Canvas, 1989. These last paintings were previously published in Cancer Stories: Creativity and Self-repair (The Analytic Press, Hillsdale NY, 1990).

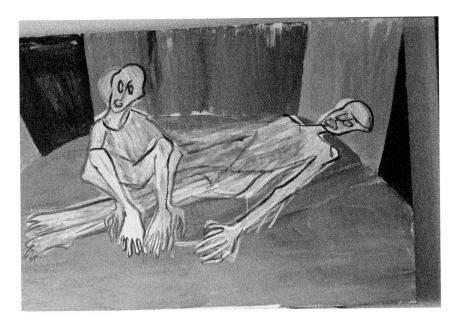

Figure 10.14 Esther Dreifuss-Kattan: "Identification," Acrylic Paint on Canvas, 1989. These last paintings were previously published in Cancer Stories: Creativity and Self-repair (The Analytic Press, Hillsdale NY, 1990).

Understanding my Wonderland-ing

Sharing my brain tumor experience

Ashley Myers-Turner and Esther Dreifuss-Kattan

Artist: Ashley Myers-Turner

One day, I was told by the UCLA communication office that a young journalist from a local public radio station was coming to the *Healing Arts* group to make a short video of the group and conduct some interviews with participants and with me for their website. I communicated to Ashley Myers-Turner, the journalist/videographer, that it would be best if she would come first without her video camera to participate in the group and get a feeling for art therapy. She could then return the following week with her video camera to interview patients.

In the "Healing Arts" group, the cancer patients first introduce themselves with a couple of sentences and discuss their medical/cancer history, after which the interns, medical students and other guests introduce themselves. When Ashley arrived to participate in the group, I asked her to introduce herself. To my surprise, Ashley mentioned that she was a recent brain cancer survivor as well as a photographer, video artist/journalist, writer, musician and a dance therapist. I was shocked and amazed that this barely 30-year-old journalist was also a cancer survivor. Ashley's manner was open, tuned to the group members' stories and the group process, and her execution of the project we did that day turned out to be very creative. She suggested that she come to my office to interview me during the week. There I learned that she had documented in self-portraits, photographs and other imagery the strange symptoms she experienced before and after being diagnosed with an astrocytoma, a type of brain tumor. She shared these pictures with her doctors as well as with friends and family. Before and after surgery, and during her recovery, Ashley transformed the trauma of seizures, mental confusion and disassociations—and her fear of these symptoms—into beautiful but uncanny digital collages. Her work owes much to her great artistic talents, acute self-perception and knowledge of brain anatomy.

These collages were not only aesthetic art pieces but also served Ashley as brain maps, allowing her to describe to her doctors her confusing symptoms before being diagnosed with brain cancer, after surgery and during her recovery. Art making also helped her familiarize herself with her new repaired self after her recovery. I asked Ashley if she would like to participate in our exhibition: "Art and Cancer: From the Canvas to the Couch," which took place a few years ago in the New Center for Psychoanalysis in Los Angeles, and she happily agreed. In the passage below, Ashley recounts her experience with her brain tumor in her own words.

Esther Dreifuss-Kattan

"Why are you giggling?" asked the urgent care doctor. He furrowed his brow with concern. I'm used to this question since I often giggle to myself, often about small things like unintentional puns or ironic happenstance. This time I was giggling out of horrifying anxiety. I also, as instructed, was carefully following the doctor's fingers with my eyes, yet my mind kept trailing off, concerned that I might fail this simple test, unsure what that would mean for my diagnosis.

"I'm just worried I'm going to fail this test," I said, owning the anxiety but not the laughter that came from it entirely.

Of course the doctor had every right to be questioning my quick change in mood, considering my cheeks were still red, blotchy and glossy with tears from just moments before. I'm sure I seemed unstable. I owed my trip to urgent care to feeling unstable, and to more: to the inexplicable smells of burnt rubber that would overpower me, to fumbling over names when I spoke as if my mouth had lost connection to my brain, and, most urgently, to the "out-of-body" experiences I kept lapsing into and the unknown voices that kept speaking to me.

"I'm going to recommend you get a brain MRI and talk to a neurologist, just to be safe," replied the doctor.

Warning: brain nerd interlude ahead. I've always thought MRIs are actually intriguingly cool. I got my undergraduate degree in Cognitive Science. I loved learning about the cortical homunculus, an image that superimposes human body parts onto the areas in the brain where the motor function of each body part is controlled. I would modify the image in my mind, imagining a series of well-defined spaces for the fingers on my left hand—created by years of scale and étude practice on my violin—and a less defined blob shape where the fingers of my right hand controlled the bow with a full team effort. I wanted to touch a brain and feel its texture. Was it rubbery, slimy and soft? Or grainy and easy to mush together? I marveled at how we could recall vivid details about miniscule moments by firing chemicals between identical monochromatic cells.

Several days after the urgent care visit I went to the MRI facility. I sat through the constant clicks, loud thuds and high-pitched squeals emitted by the machine for 40 minutes and happily walked out with portraits of my very own brain. Unfortunately, I still had to wait a couple of weeks before I met with my neurologist who could tell me what these images actually revealed. I remember feeling annoyed that I didn't know enough about the brain to read the scan and nervous about the secrets the scan film contained (Figure 7.1).

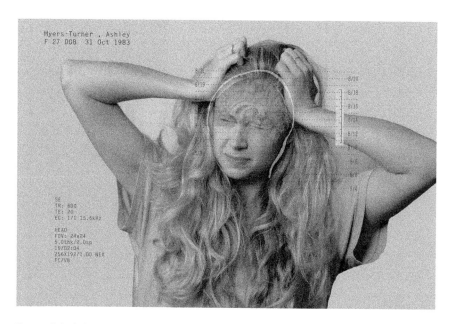

Figure 7.1 Ashley Myers-Turner, "Untitled I," Digital Photography and MRI, 2011.

To keep myself busy while I waited for my follow-up appointment, I decided to explore the scan, attempting to further understand this inner space of mine, to somehow connect it with my outside, and, in the process, maybe coax the scan to trust me and spill its brain guts!

To aid in this exploration, I set up a camera to take some self-portraits. This was back before the WiFi camera app boom, so I jury-rigged a wired system connected to my laptop for image visibility and used a mixture of self-timer and adept toe-to-keyboard manipulation to take the shots. I matched the placement of my head to the anatomical scans, moving my head by centimeters up, down, left and right. I tried to be patient and exacting, but detail-focused technical work has never been my strength. Hundreds of frames later, unsure if I had anything usable at all, I finally let go of the details. I let go of the spatial placement. I let go of the exacting attitude. I let go of the hard exterior science and instead took a handful of photos focused on my felt experience during this waiting period: frustration, confusion, physical pain, emotional chaos. And in these frames I finally felt relief from my anxiety.

After shooting the photos, I spent the next few days delving into Photoshop to combine the MRI image with my self-portrait photos. As opposed to the feelings of constraint and frustration I fought while shooting specified angles, working on the details of this new image felt more exploratory and free. And the final product emerged like an authentic expression of my current state—a divided but united, stressed-out test subject, circling in a holding pattern before the storm, yearning to be a continuous whole.

Finally sitting in the office of my new neurologist, with all his diplomas and honorary certificates proudly displayed on the walls, I stumbled over my words attempting to explain the event that caused me to visit urgent care to begin with (Figure 7.2).

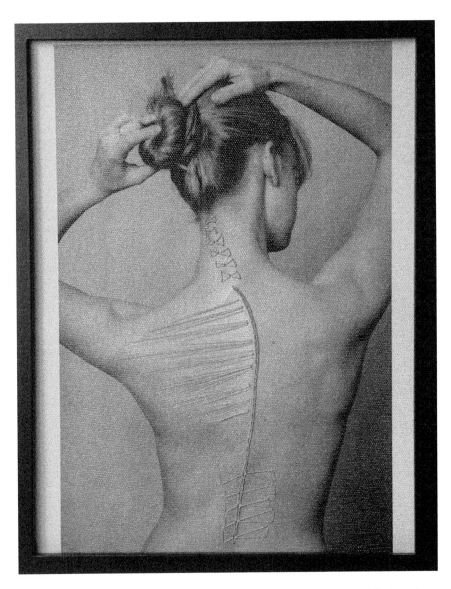

Figure 7.2 Ashley Myers-Turner, "Spine," Digital Photography and Embroidery, 2012 Embroidery.

It had been a hot late summer day, and I was sitting at my computer writing an email. I felt this creeping sensation up my back that consumed my shoulders. I started to smell burning rubber. My vision blurred. Seconds stretched into minutes and seemingly into hours, yet none of these measures had any meaning because time no longer existed. I felt myself rise from my body and hover just over my shoulder. I watched my body continue typing gibberish into the email. And I had a thought assuring my now flowing self that I could be released from this body: "let her take it, I don't need it anymore." I could let it go, knowing it's being taken care of. Suddenly I once again inhabited my body, still typing away, the same commercial still playing on the TV.

While I was worried that this sounded crazy, my neurologist took this description in stride, not missing a beat. Apparently I was having seizures. Not seizures as I had known them. No convulsions. No tics. No uncontrollable urination or incontinence. Instead, I was having complex partial seizures that only affected part of my brain and resulted in this personal, internal experience, all the while concealing its drastic alterations of my consciousness from others (Figure 7.3).

So my brain *did* have a secret!

This first seizure experience made a lasting, visually vivid impression on me. I tried to explain it to family and friends, and while they nodded and said they understood, I felt there was still a communication barrier between my experience and their understanding. Once again I picked up my camera,

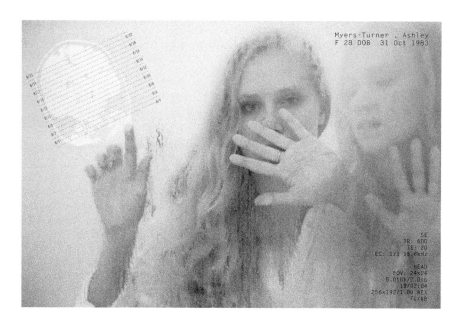

Figure 7.3 Ashley Myers-Turner, "Untitled 2," Digital Photography and MRI, 2011.

as I had with my MRI scans, in an attempt to create a visual that would break down that barrier. And once again, the process of creating this image allowed me to further explore a similar divide, the relationship, or gap, between myself and my brain, making the experience less foreign and more a part of my identity.

I was referred to a neurosurgeon who told me I had a cancerous brain tumor that was causing the seizures. Later that month he opened my skull and removed a small astrocytoma tumor from the left amygdala, leaving me with some titanium plate party favors and a very long recovery hangover.

Brain surgery recovery touches each person differently. My recovery felt like an adolescent experimenting with drugs. The room would spin. I felt like I was flying. My furniture would spontaneously move and morph into different shapes.

One day my supervisor at work was sending me out to cover a breaking news story and wanted to ensure I had fresh batteries for my voice recorder. With a battery strength tester he went through a pile of batteries separating the fully charged from the dead. I had to bite my lip to not giggle (I was getting a lot of practice covering inappropriate giggles). Looking at the batteries, my only thought was: "Get rid of those evil villains. I'm only taking the Supermans!" which nonsense was extra funny to me considering I had never followed comic book superheroes and couldn't name a single Superman villain (Figure 7.4).

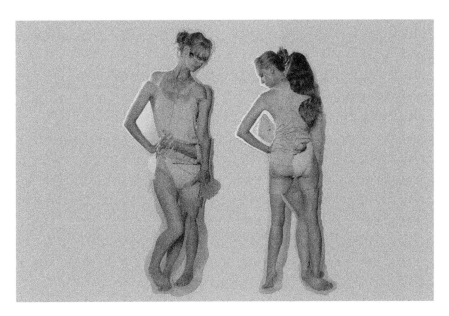

Figure 7.4 Ashley Myers-Turner, "Ashley in Wonderland," Digital Collage, 2011.

While I was taking medication to control the seizures, exhaustion or anxiety would sometimes trigger a new symptom. One day I would feel like my fingers were growing too fat to clasp my hands together. Or the room was growing larger, myself smaller, leaving me searching for Alice's "drink me" bottle as I fell into Wonderland.

At this time all I could do to bridge my inner and outer worlds was continue to create images. I collected images from the physical world—graffiti walls, book references, my MRI scans—and manipulated them to match my felt experience. I shared these pieces with friends and family, hoping they would be open and understanding to my strange experiences and continue to support me, while I balanced my body and brain into a unified and whole composition again (Figure 7.5).

Now, nearly four years since surgery, my brain and I have learned to communicate. I rarely experience seizures. While I'm prone to migraines, I'm armed with tools to relieve the pain. I visit my oncologist multiple times each year to look at new MRI scans. And during the physical exam I still giggle during the eye test.

My art making continues, but at a less unremitting pace. During a recent chat with a group of cancer survivors who also make art related to their diagnosis, the discussion turned to the time frame of art creation. Several people mentioned that their art making came after the event of the diagnosis, once there had been time to breathe and process. This seemed like a consensus for the rest of the group, so my silence on the topic attracted attention. I had to explain that waiting for space before processing through art is completely counterintuitive for me. With my own health history, the event inspired the art and I relied on the art exercise to help me process the event. The art needed to happen as close to the event and my subsequent reaction as possible in order to be useful for me.

With fewer physical symptoms these days, I have found myself wading through a completely new set of issues common to the young adult cancer community. I feel almost splintered in two. A diagnosis with treatment and recovery forces a suspension, letting friends and colleagues continue to move forward in life, defining their place in the world, while I find myself in a holding pattern. Defining myself along any of their lines or narratives came at a prohibitive cost when I was in an *Alice in Wonderland* haze. I was faced with the question of how to prepare for typical life events—marriage, kids, retirement—when an atypical life event might kill me before I get there.

On the other side, I did follow a career trajectory. I underwent defining experiences and developed characteristics and memories that have made me a unique person. But brain surgery tampered with my memory, reorganized my priorities, shifted my point of view. I don't remember all the events that have defined my self. Will anyone understand my new point of view and new priorities? Will my friends and family still recognize me? Sometimes it feels

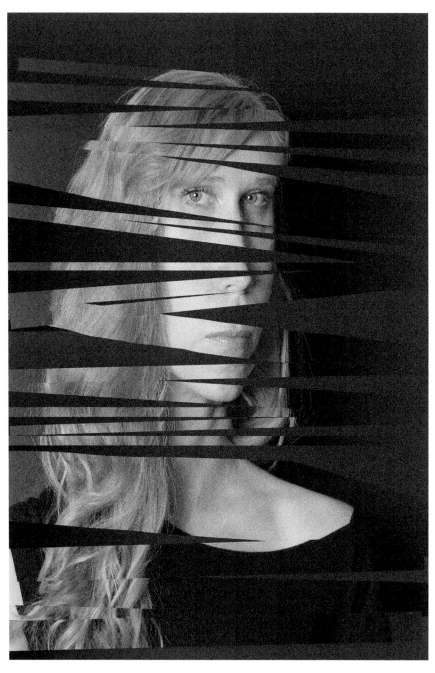

Figure 7.5 Ashley Myers-Turner, "Split Head I," Digital Photography, 2011.

as though a part of me has been erased and I'm still waiting on an updated snapshot to fill in the blanks.

In 2011, in the catalog of the "Art and Cancer: From the Canvas to the Couch" exhibition at the New Center for Psychoanalysis in Los Angeles, Ashley wrote:

> Through this process, I have relied on my photography and art to help me reach an increased level of comfort with my diagnosis. Through my images, I have specifically explored some of my physical symptoms, such as disrupted body awareness, head-rupturing migraines, nausea-inducing vertigo, and disorienting neural activity. I have asked myself the questions: "How am I am pieced and sewn together? How do my physical and mental self-images interact?" Even though I've lived and experienced my brain through my life, I had never actually seen my brain until I looked at my recent MRI images. The fusing of my self-portraits with my MRI images also allows me to try to accept this strange looking, malfunctioning, imperfect brain as part of me.
>
> While it has been three years since my surgery, and many of the most intense symptoms have subsided, I am still exploring my body, brain and self and their connection to each other through my art
>
> (Myers-Tuner, 2011)

Theoretical reflections

Esther Dreifuss-Kattan

While creating her collages the artist confronted her new catastrophic reality straight on. Ashley was able to transform her traumatic event with its fragmentation and alteration of perceptions into strong, generatively layered collages. The artist looked through the lens of her camera and at her digitized images of her brain in an attempt to track her traumatic symptoms. She found, through her creative process, a new integration of self, a novel presence, as well as tried to recover was not there, her ghostly, altered self. (Crimp, 1980). Ashley's photographic image externalized her inner discourse and emphasized her singularity as she became both subject and object in her art, providing coherence and exposing her inwardness (Krauss, 1984). Like one looking into a mirror, she contemplated her otherness and also her resemblance to these images, trying to understand her new and shocking identity as a woman who has a brain tumor. Ashley envisioned her potential future as a patient as perhaps only an artist could, paying special attention to the overlap of reality and phantasm, and seeking to represent the actual experience of the present in conjunction with her former life as a whole and healthy person. Through the power of the digital collage medium to express two representations at once, Ashley was able to disrupt the overwhelming force of her trauma, focusing on her wish to survive while also accessing her otherness (Caruth, 1996). Her imagery overlaid both conscious and unconscious ideations of self and other, of fear and medical pathology, while tapping into her frightening bodily experiences. By looking at the imagery, we the viewers could see inside her head and thus know—but also do not know—her new experience of her present self and her experience, while sick, of the idea of a healthy other. These self-portrait digital photo collages allowed the artist to play with her multiple self-perceptions in an attempt to explore and accept her new but imperfect wholeness.

Artistic expression in the face of medical trauma allowed Ashley to convert disturbing bodily symptoms that threatened the integrity of her self, turning their meaning away from death and closer to *jouissance* (Lacan, 1972). Ashley's desire for creative self-representation in order to communicate her new confusing medical, cognitive and psychological symptoms also helped her to maintain the restoration of self, in spite of life threat (Apollon, 2012). This life force, with its deep cultural and artistic enjoyment, reinforced her identity as an artist who wanted to live.

By showing us her very private imagery, Ashley hoped to escape social isolation and psychological detachment. As an analogy, we remember that if we believe that the ego can be formed in the mirror stage, when the baby discovers herself in the mirror or is mirrored in the mother's or significant other's face, then we see how a visual superimposition or equivalency between the other and itself is vital to the ego, even though the other is perceived as altered. Ashley found a similar equivalency through the lens of her camera and her expressive powers, between her altered self and the new other self. Fusing them in her collages into an integrated composition or new form, communicating the authenticity of her pictorial testimony. (Benjamin, 1968. According to Bollas (1987), parents help their baby by facilitating the transition from early private, enigmatic personal expression like babbling into a more real language structure, thus creating the first transformational object, allowing the baby to venture away from the mother while remaining verbally connected. Ashley used her multiple, creative digital self-portraits to transform her own frightening, fragmenting physical experiences with her malignant brain trauma and her temporary loss of control over her brain activity and body coordination into transformational objects with their own comprehensible language and strong aesthetic. Playing with different photographic multiple identities, stitched and sewn together in both digital and material ways, she searched for her old self while she created her new self at the same time. Her images show physical regression as well as new integration, moving from her very private realm of self-expression toward the outside, as well as toward culture and the world at large.

These self-portrait digital photo collages have a distinct origin in particular coordinates of time and space and are connected to Ashley's particular cancer journey. Her photographs can take the form of digital manipulations and of print reproductions overlaid with her brain scans, enlarged, and collaged with threads and lights. As Ashley's specific experiences modulate how these works function as her testimony, we as viewers and readers are invited to observe with what Susan Sontag calls an "ethic of seeing," taking the camera to be the "ideal arm" of Ashley's "consciousness in its acquisitive mood" (Sontag, 1977, p. 81). The artist, in other words, allows her symptoms and fears to surface in these works for all of us to see and to elicit our empathy with her; she stages an intimate encounter, almost a merging, of the self-as-photographer and the self-as-subject. Of course, as intimacy's mood can shift, so can its proximity become invasive, allowing the tone of these works' photographic disclosure of Ashley's self to change from vulnerable to paranoid or even aggressive. Photography can excerpt very specific, frozen slices of time from life, snapshots of the wide variety of emotions and transitory considerations Ashley went through while faced with her mortality. As Cartier-Bresson (1999) says in *The Mind's Eye*: "Photographic reportage is to stay engaged with the subject ... for me the camera is a sketchbook, an instrument of intuition and spontaneity" (https://www.magnumphotos.com/arts-culture/art/the-minds-eye/). For Ashley, photographing herself is like a sketchbook, an artistic diary of the status of her brain and mind and of its extreme distortions and regressions, effects which provoked terror of new symptoms.

In the introduction to the French literary theorist, critic and philosopher Roland Barthes's book *Camera Lucida: Reflection On Photography*, Geoff Dyer quotes an interview with Barthes from 1977 in which he claims that "the photographer bears witness essentially to his own subjectivity" in a sort of indexical relation (Dyer, 2010, p. xi). For Barthes, a photograph was not only a record of something now absent that was present in "reality in a past state"; nor is it a record of "what has been" or what Lacan calls alternately the *touché*, the encounter, the *occasion* or the Real. Rather, a photograph is a subtle moment in which the photographer tells the truth. The photographer's "second sight" does not only consist solely of *seeing*, but rather of *being there*. (Barthes, p. 47). Regarding the distinction between the two, Barthes recounts an anecdote in which the Czech poet Gustav Janouch told Franz Kafka that "the necessary condition for an image is sight," who replied, smiling: "we photograph things in order to drive them out of our own minds. My stories are a way of shutting my eyes" (Barthes, p. 53). I believe both Janouch's plain sight and Kafka's blissful oblivion serve as motivations for Ashley's photography: she did want to communicate her symptoms to her health professionals and close family members, but at the same time took refuge from their terror by externalizing them. Her photographs mean both being there, in Barthes' words, and being mercifully distant.

As a summary, we can say the art-therapeutic mirror stage of photography confronts illness while offering respite from it, oftentimes all in the same work or a single set of images. "The photograph of the missing being," says Susan Sontag, "will touch me like the delayed rays of a star." (Barthes, p. 81). Because her experience of mortality dilates in time or shows a prolonged threat of dying, Ashley's case displaces the usual conflation of a "missing being" with a deceased one, as we all know from looking at a photograph of a partner, friend, parent or grandparent who has died. Ashley's "missing being" becomes, conversely, her old, healthy sense of the integration of her physical self. Though the camera is, in this way, a tool with which to diagnose and elucidate the patient's unique experience of loss, it also opens unknown potentials of imagination and creativity, leading to a sort of playground and resting place for the Ashley to engage in her characteristic task of finding new equivalencies between inner and outer reality. The aesthetic fluidity between the photographer's self and the Other, between self-presentation and representation, can reflect and express a realm of personal and creative tension within the photographer.

A set of photographs or self-portraits also creates an archive, a site to remember the past as both happy and traumatic. In *Archive Fever* (1996), Jacques Derrida observes that the archive addresses the chronic impulse to collect, keep and order material. It also, for Derrida, speaks with a distinct voice of authority and presents a compulsion to attend to mortality. Where artists and photographers generally use the pictorial archive to connect images, in our case, the archive offers a timeline of life from a cancer diagnosis through treatment and recovery, stringing together memories, feelings and symptoms, exploring the recent presence of illness and resolving in the immediate past of renewed health and well-being. The images and fragments of memories in the digital archive are there for the artist as she reconsiders them to be a reflection of her biographical past, as much as they might also conserve pieces of history or contemporary culture within an aesthetic time capsule. The digital photographic archive Ashley preserves on her website hosts these historical and personal narratives, prompting the re-constellation of a past not necessarily understood at the time, or now, and furnishing this material as a kind of re-narration that tests the ways the past can be reformed in a temporal "synchronicity." These reconfigurations provide the photographer with her own personal aesthetic of illness and recovery that she can share with family and friends, as well as with strangers and a wider culture. Not unlike psychoanalysis, this personal photographic, pictorial database not only aims at the preservation of our or other historic "pasts" but also facilitates a rethinking of her past, an actual re-formulation of this past in a creative and dynamic way. "Pastness," or the past that is relived, re-experienced and reorganized in the present all over again, can thus be better metabolized psychologically (Bettkelly-Chalmers, 2016).

Images

1   *Diagnosis—2011*, Photography and Digital MRI
    "Diagnosis" was created to reflect complicated feelings of helplessness during my diagnosis of complex partial seizures that led to a diagnosis of brain cancer.
2   *Seizure—2011*, Photography and Digital MRI
    "Seizure" depicts an out-of-body experience felt during a partial complex seizure. This seizure experience led me to seek help from urgent care.
3   *Ashley in Wonderland—2012*, Photography
    "Ashley in Wonderland" illustrated my experience with Alice In Wonderland syndrome (aka Todd's syndrome), which affects perception by distorting size and shape of the body and other objects. This syndrome is usually associated with migraines and brain tumors.
4   *Aura—2013*, photography on canvas with embroidery
    Before a seizure I sometimes experience an aura. For me this is a warning sign. Sometimes a seizure follows, but sometimes the aura is all I feel. Often my auras include a feeling that runs up my spine and spreads over my shoulders.

References

Apollon, W. (2002). The Letter of the Body. In R. Hughes and K.R. Malone (Eds.), *After Lacan, Clinical Practice and the Subject of the Unconscious* (pp. 103–116). Albany: SUNY Press.

Barthes, R. (2010). *Camera Lucida: Reflections on Photography* (R. Howard, Trans.). New York: Hill and Wang.

Benjamin, W. (1968). The Work of Art in the Age of Mechanical Reproduction. In *Illuminations: Essays and Reflections* (pp. 217–251). London: Harcourt.

Bettkelly-Chalmers, K. (2016). *Beyond the Clock: The Aesthetics of Time in Contemporary Art* (Thesis). Retrieved from Research Repository, University of Auckland, New Zealand. http://hdl.handle.net/2292/28799.

Bollas, C. (1987). *The Shadow of The Object*. New York: Columbia University Press.

Cartier-Bresson, H. (1999). *The Mind's Eye: Writings on Photography and Photographers*. New York: Aperture Foundation.

Caruth, K. (1996). *Unclaimed Experience, Trauma, Narrative, and History*. Baltimore, MD: Johns Hopkins University Press.

Crimp, D. (1980). The Photographic Activity of Postmodernism. *October, 15* (15), 91–101.

Derrida, J. (1998). *Archive Fever*. Chicago, IL: University of Chicago Press.

Dyer, Geoff. (2010). "Foreword" to Roland Barthes, *Camera Lucida: Reflections on Photography* (R. Howard, Trans.). New York: Hill and Wang.

Janouch, G. (1968/1971). *Conversation with Kafka*, translated by Rees, G.; *A New Direction Book*. Frankfurt-am-Main: Fisher Verlag.

Kraus, R. (1984). A Note on Photography and the Simulacral. *October, 31* (31), 49–68.

Lacan, J. (1960). *Archive Fever: A Freudian Impression* (E. Prenowiz, Trans.). Chicago, IL: University of Chicago Press.

Lacan, J. (1972–1973). *On Feminine Sexuality the Limits of Love and Knowledge: The Seminars of Jacques Lacan, Book XX Encore* (J.-A. Miller, Ed.). New York: Norton, 1998.

Myers-Turner, A. (2011). *From the Canvas to the Couch: Art and Cancer Catalogue.* Los Angeles, CA: Shuttterfly Web Publisher.

Sontag, S. (1977). *On Photography.* New York: Picador.

Chapter 8

Cancer! Life is going on anyway and not "Cancery" enough: from track pants to yoga pants

Fighting melanoma with paper cutouts and comic books

Mary E. Walter and Esther Dreifuss-Kattan

Artist: Mary E. Walter

Fighting cancer with paper cutouts

Mary E. Walter

I was diagnosed with melanoma (skin cancer) in March 2009. While recovering from the surgery on my leg, I started attending the "Cancer and Creativity" support group that met weekly in Santa Monica. "Cancer and Creativity" rekindled my long-dormant love for art making. It also provided a way of sorting out all the conflicts, fears and frustrations of my cancer healing process.

I remember my very first day at the Creativity and Cancer Support Group. The subject was raw and unclear. I had never done this kind of art before, always preferring drawing. The colored construction paper was put on the table and it looked good. I just picked it up and started to work. Art therapy was new to me. Here is my collage (Figure 8.1):

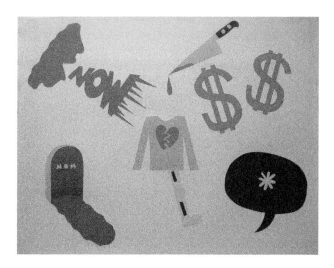

Figure 8.1 Mary E. Walter: "My Immediate Family," color construction paper on Bristol paper, 2009.

1   **MY IMMEDIATE FAMILY**, June 9, 2009, color construction paper on Bristol paper, 19″ × 24″

Each image is a symbol representing one member of my family including me. I was mourning the loss of the relationships in my family, most of all my relationship with my mom. My heart was broken. How much more loss could I take? The previous year had been the worst in my life. Making this collage, I had the feeling of each member of my immediate family encircling me. My older sister needed to get the family business done: NOW! She had to move our elderly parents closer to her where they could receive better care. When I tried to prepare our parents' house for moving, my mentally ill younger sister attempted to kill me, and that still left a sharp cloud of fear hanging over me. My brother talked of nothing but inheritances and money, amid the deep recession that had just hit the country. And the silence of my dad, who had sunk deeper into dementia, was disturbing. My yellow leg, with two raw gashes, stared back at me; this one leg harbored my melanoma and thus was the focus of my attention. Will I have to fear the rest of my life that there is more cancer lurking, undiscovered, hidden, ready to strike when I least expect it? I am now constantly vigilant and like a soldier, stiff and upright, standing on guard.

My leg was not healing well from the melanoma surgery a few months before my first "Cancer and Creativity" class and I was realizing that the persistent pain there was nerve damage that would never go away. It felt like all this fear and uncertainty surrounded me with no place to escape. Since I had never done anything like this kind of art before, I was surprised at what I created. I liked cutting out the construction paper and gluing it down, quickly and haphazardly, like arts and crafts time when I was a child. I felt free using the scissors and paper.

Maybe I used the cutout technique since a part of my leg was cut out, and my previous, stable life had been cut out for now as well; my relationships with my siblings had been cut out and had changed, and then the cutting out of my cancer by the surgeon. I like the primary colors, the sharp edges and the basic shapes against the white background.

I felt safe to make art together in the group with all the other cancer artists who had gone through the trauma of a cancer diagnosis and its treatment. I put my picture away after the class, after we looked at it together, and I didn't show it to anyone else outside the group. All the images are ordinary objects, but they are arranged around me and have great significance. There was so much physical and psychological pain in my life at that time; much of it was my family trauma on top of a cancer diagnosis.

Some thoughts

Esther Dreifuss-Kattan

I remember the day when Mary walked into the Cancer and Creativity group for the first time. She came a little late and the twelve participants and I were sitting around four very large tables that formed a big square. The patients were in the process of telling their fellow group members and me how their week was going, and recounting their health and life problems. It was a very inclusive group, mostly women and one man at different ages with different cancers in different stages, and some were cancer survivors. Mary sat down at the end; after everybody had spoken, she tried to summarize what seemed a rather traumatic period in her life. Not only was it just a few months after Mary's melanoma surgery on her leg, living with the fear that surgery might have caused permanent damage and pain, but she also delved into some disturbing experiences with her family: a mentally ill sibling and a mother who had recently died, and the beginning of dementia in her aging father. Due to her cancer surgery she had stopped working as a special effects editor. This professional leave of absence seemed a relief for Mary, as her type of job is very intense, demanding long hours and night work to meet Hollywood deadlines. But being out of work also meant less money; and if the recovery either physically and psychologically took too long, her employer's health insurance would lapse.

Looking at her very skillfully done collage in colored construction and tissue paper, we see the urgency of each of the family events she describes above in their singularity. The blue face of the older sister is screaming *Now*, with sharp blue spikes penetrating the space at the top of the page. We see equally powerfully rendered her mother's tombstone, with its fresh brown dirt attesting to the acuteness of the loss. A big sharp bloody knife still dripping testifies to the scary assault of her younger sister, who attacked Mary when she was cleaning out their parents' house to sell it. This was necessary to allow her father to live closer to her older sister on the west coast who could take care of him. The green dollar signs loom like the financial uncertainty for Mary and her other two siblings, or the greed of her brother's threatening to scoop up their parents' savings. Then, wearing a pink shirt with a broken heart on it, one leg missing entirely, while the yellow leg seems taped up in two places to cover up wounds, is part of a figure representing Mary herself. A nearly empty black speech bubble on the right side shows the little star sign we find on our phones. Maybe Mary asks herself who can dial time back, to a sane and healthy past without loss? Each piece of the collage is perfectly rendered in strong and beautiful colors, in a very detailed and balanced manner. Only Mary, without a head, with no hands and leaning on one sick leg is totally off kilter, physically and emotionally.

Indeed, Mary's other problems are not suddenly erased because she has cancer now. Mary's recent past was overwhelming, and she had no time to address her different traumata before her very malignant cancer struck. At the same time, we see in the strong colors and balanced composition some humor, a flash of irony that intimates Mary has the capacity, with help of her creativity and art therapy, to work through her distress, and will eventually find her footing again (Figure 8.2).

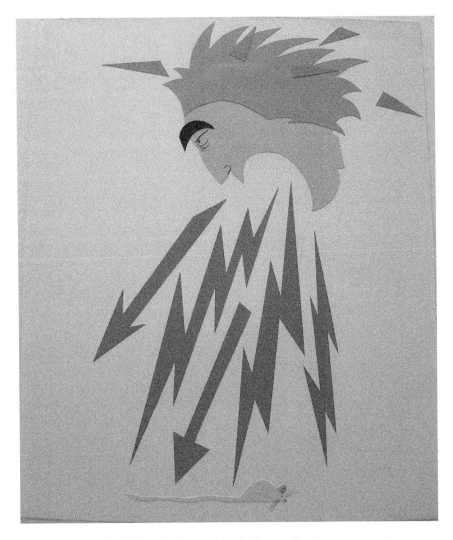

Figure 8.2 Mary E. Walter: "Please Call Me Doctor," color construction paper, graphite pencil on Bristol paper, 2010.

Mary Walter

2   **PLEASE CALL ME, DOCTOR!** May 25, 2010, color construction paper, graphite pencil on Bristol paper, 14" × 17"

A doctor had promised that he would call with the results of some follow-up tests to the melanoma surgery and never did. I was growing more angry and terrified as one assistant told me that the doctor would need to speak to me personally, and she was not allowed to give me the results of the test. I wanted to unleash a torrent of wrath on the medical establishment, hoping they would feel as frightened as I was feeling.

I am represented in the picture as the shouting, disembodied head, realizing that I wanted the doctor to feel like the mouse below. My anger and fear are the red bolts and arrows. My hair is really brown, but I could only find orange paper that day and I thought it a great choice of color to express feelings of rage. My eyes' expression feels distant and not focused on the mouse-doctor, with lots of rage and anger spouting out of me in all directions.

I started out wanting to express how frightened I was at the possibility of the melanoma returning, but when I was finished, the art revealed more of the rage I felt about my melanoma and its treatment that I could not express verbally. Other cancer patients and survivors in the group knew immediately what this picture was about when they saw the title. The anxiety and even panic of waiting for test results is very common to anyone who has suffered a life-threatening disease. So is the extreme anger and rage that hides the fear and anxiety when for waiting for the results.

In retrospect, looking at this piece now, a few years later, it brings back all that rage and anger. I realize that I felt like the mouse too, small and frightened. It seemed that all the trauma and horrible experiences of that year had reduced me to an insignificant creature that could be crushed at any moment for no reason. The burden of carrying the cancer and family trauma weakened me to a state of fragility that I thought could break any time. I wondered if I could carry on under the constant barrage of fear, hypervigilance and physical pain. I wanted to hide like a little mouse.

Some thoughts

Esther Dreifuss-Kattan

Mary once again here used her amazing skill with paper cutouts. The title I suggested for this picture of that particular day was "Speaking Up." The title derives from an issue brought up by the group members who were discussing how difficult it is to make one's voice heard with oncologists: how intimidating it can be for them to speak up when having a request, a question or confusion over what the doctor had communicated.

Mary illustrated her own head with flaming orange hair that sprouted words shown as red arrows. The arrows grow big, flying toward the tiny yellow mouse. I pointed out to Mary that what really seems to have happened in this picture was that a powerful doctor was shooting red arrows of contempt at her, who had turned in horror into a tiny, toxic-looking mouse. Not being heard or taken seriously by the doctor can diminish patients, who are already very vulnerable because of cancer and it treatments. Even though we are all rationally aware that doctors can be overwhelmed—working too many hours with too many patients, and also having to wait till they receive the pathology back from the laboratory—the cancer patients' fear overrides all realistic expectations. The bigger the hospital is, moreover, the harder it is to actually locate the right doctor at a given time or even a trusted nurse, aggravating psychic bewilderment with physical isolation.

The ambivalence of Mary's picture is a striking characteristic. Cancer and cancer treatment can make anybody angry and impatient, and since the doctor is the one in charge, all is projected onto her. On the other hand, cancer makes you very timid and vulnerable, even as patience wears thin and vulnerability sparks into anger. Artistic expression and psychotherapy is a good way to become aware of both the potential for rage at, as well as the need for a close, empathic relationship with your treating oncologist. Together with other cancer patients, one can find a way to approach one's doctor and explain one's personal need and fears. If such a rapprochement seems unlikely to work, one might have a good reason to get a second opinion from another doctor, and to clarify one's medical and psychological need. The patient too can come to realize he or she needs to find another doctor that has more of a capacity to be empathic and supportive when diagnosing a recurrence of illness, one who understands patients' frustration and spikes in anxiety and does not take it too personally. Mary addressed the patient doctor relationship in another of her pictures, entitled "That's Easy," that is not reproduced (Figure 8.3).

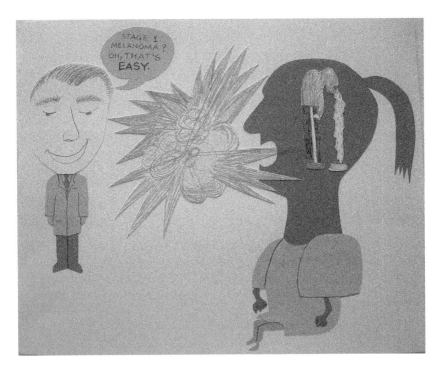

Figure 8.3 Mary E. Walter: "That's Easy," color construction paper, colored pencil on Bristol paper, 2010.

Mary Walter, on "That's Easy"

My assignment was to think of and express a conversation I would like to initiate or could imagine with somebody. An off-handed comment by a new oncologist I was seeing sent me into a rage. In the picture, everything is floating with nothing to connect to. It shows two people with very different experiences of cancer. I felt disconnected and adrift. Neither one of us seemed to be hearing what the other was saying. While I was scared of my cancer and tried to explain something to the doctor, he was in his mind with the next patient already, looking longingly at the door.

I told this oncologist of the nerve damage and the leg pain that I was experiencing, but he brushed it off and reacted to my visit as if I had made a mistake. "Who told you to see me? Why are you wasting my time? You are all better now, there is no reason to come back!" His reaction was the complete opposite of what I had been told by my previous surgeon. I was frustrated and angry, but didn't know how to direct these feelings; I was able to manage or work through them in my artistic expression, however, and thus felt protected in the art therapy group by artists who had experienced similar experiences with their doctors (Figure 8.4).

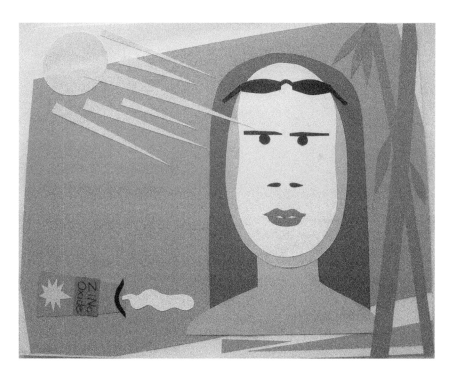

Figure 8.4 Mary E. Walter: "Kabuki? Noh? Sunscreen Mask," color construction paper, Felt Marker on Bristol, 2010.

Mary Walter

3   **KABUKI? NOH?... SUNSCREEN MASK**, Aug. 31, 2010, color construction paper, felt maker on Bristol paper, 14″ × 17″

One day as I was performing my daily ritual of applying sunscreen, I noticed I looked like an actor in the makeup or masks of the *kabuki* and *noh* Japanese theatre. I feel the threatening spikes of sunlight daily and the damage it could do to create another melanoma. The next time I was in art therapy group, the cutout papers seemed a perfect way to render the ghostlike features that the sunscreen mask created.

I find the task of putting on sunscreen every day a disgusting chore. It's so thick and greasy and I feel I am being sealed in for the day, putting on my mask in order to face the world. I wanted to show a typical beautiful Southern California day with all the trappings of good health and good times for some people. For me, I look out and see the sun beating down and think of how I will defend myself against the UV rays that can cause another skin cancer. And there is also the thought lingering in the back of my mind that perhaps the materials that make up sunscreen could be causing some other toxic disease that has not been discovered yet. All these thoughts are an expression of the acute anxiety I felt about my melanoma returning.

Noh masks have these wonderful smudged eyebrows that are a straight line. *Kabuki* makeup has severe lines that enhance the actor's skill. I daily go out into the world in my mask, though when the zinc oxide has been absorbed into my skin mine becomes invisible to all but myself. It just feels like a thick, molten mask when I am out in that sunshine. I like the sun, but hate the sunscreen. It's funny, isn't it?

Some thoughts

Esther Dreifuss-Kattan

As Mary came once a week to the "Cancer and Creativity" group she made friends and felt more competent in her art making. She shared her issues both verbally and in her art with the group members and me. As she healed physically, her humor suddenly surfaced and her art making became more playful. Even though sunscreen now reminded her every day of her vulnerability to melanoma, despite how her leg was healing and tests came back negative, her association to the Japanese theatre shows a lot of creativity and imagination, turning an ugly and annoying necessity into fun and pleasant imagery. The sticky sunscreen becomes an actor's makeup and persona, leading to a creative transformation. The mood and facial expression of the actor is hidden by the mask and she can take on any role that corresponds to the predrawn mask. For Mary she cannot forget yet that she used to have melanoma because it is too early and she has to protect herself from the sun. She can choose to show a happy face that is not always real, as it is hidden below the surface, but eventually when the time and place are right it will shine through, as in this colorful collage with its impressive details and humor. Donning this mask is also one of the few strategies for control that remain to Mary to direct her future: putting on a hat when going into the sun and protecting her skin from another melanoma with heavy, greasy sunscreen.

Mary Walter

I have always been attracted to printmaking. In my picture "POV OF MY GIMPY LEG" (no reproduction), I used some nice pieces of cardboard sitting around the room where we would meet for the art therapy session. I decided to attempt making an Andy Warhol–type print using the cardboard as the mechanism for stamping alternate colors of paint. For me, yellow represents sickness, disease and infection. Red is blood.

Making this piece, I felt lazy and thought that rather than cut out many different-colored legs, it would be easier to just print them out. Little did I know how difficult it would be to carefully cut the cardboard into the shape I wanted and then to get the paint to lay down evenly on the paper. I liked the hole that was left when I was done cutting the form of the leg. The cutting of the cardboard started to remind me of my own surgery and how it left a deep wound, a positive and negative space. What is lost: a hole; what is gained: made whole. Something was removed and transformed the architecture of my whole body, causing some imbalance. The resulting pain in my hip reminded me of the Bible story of when Jacob wrestled with the angel that represented God. I felt that I had also wrestled with God through this rough period of my life of cancer and family trauma.

As with my surgery, I felt like I had a need to peel the top layer off some of the cardboard forms to see what would be revealed underneath. The melanoma tumor had invaded a lower level of skin that then had to be removed. This is my POV (point of view), to use a cinematic term. If the viewer looks at it, it seems to be a right leg. But it is not. This is what I see when *I* look down at my left leg, not what someone else sees (Figure 8.5).

4   **LAST DAY OF ART THERAPY**, April 24, 2012, tissue paper & fabric on Bristol paper, 19″ × 24″

I had never been able to master painting but found I could manipulate and make some softer edges with the gluing-down of tissue paper. It could also be folded over many times to make many of the same images from only one cut, like making paper dolls. Tearing the images can bring surprises.

I went to the very last day of this art therapy group with a very heavy heart. I had spent a few years with my fellow cancer survivors. Many of my

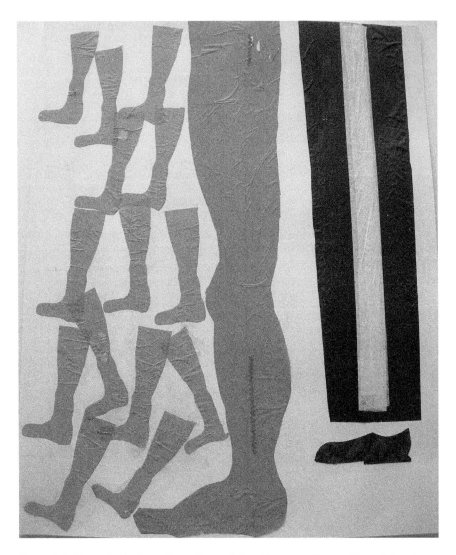

Figure 8.5 Mary E. Walter: "Last Day of Art Therapy: Tissue Paper," fabric on Bristol paper, 2012.

new friends had died. We had all gone through the terror of tests and X-rays and scans, and the fearful waiting for results and follow-ups to our cancers. Many tears had been shed. Many milestones celebrated. I came into the group without having made any art for many, many years and came out with a renewed enthusiasm for my first love, art making. My fellow participants had listened patiently to me, as I had to them. It was safe in the group to be vulnerable as well as scared. Tissue paper is also fragile and hard to work with once glued down. It tears easily and the colors bleed. It can be layered many times to be transparent or opaque and it wrinkles fast.

This group helped me to stand on my two legs again. I came in wearing track pants, but my fellow patients made it safe for me to expose my wounds and myself. I mourned all my losses with this group and shared and was encouraged by others and my friends. I found myself looking forward to each of our weekly meetings. Making art with all these new friends transformed my life. It brought forth healing and was an outlet for many feeling and thoughts I did not know how to express verbally. It brought me back to my inner core, my creative, artistic self. Track pants are a symbol of the only way I could find comfort as I struggled to heal my leg. The pink leg with rickrack scars is how I was able to be vulnerable and open in the safety of the containing "Cancer and Creativity" therapy group. The many green legs are the group and its leader, Esther, and the new life they gave me by listening without judgment as I entered a new, healthier part of my life. I am now back at my work in the film industry. The film I worked on most recently is nominated for an Oscar!

Mary Walter: Introduction

Not "Cancery" enough: from track pants to yoga pants

I stumbled upon a class about creating comic books taught by Jim Higgins at Meltdown Comics in Hollywood at the same time that I started the Cancer and Creativity group with Esther in Santa Monica, a perfect collision of worlds.

I went to art school in New York City, majoring in graphic design and fashion illustration, but then most of my working life has been in the Hollywood film industry in various capacities as a visual effects technician, camera assistant and assistant editor. The majority of motion pictures are viewed at 24 frames per second; I always loved watching the small changes that occurred from frame to frame on the editing equipment, either analog or digital. But that medium's often formulaic tableaux, thinly disguised and clichéd, lost their sheen many years ago for me.

Maybe because I had spent so much time looking at motion picture images, one frame at a time, laid out on a light box and in the company of professional storytellers, I got interested in arranging the individual images, the "frames" of a comic book called "panels," that can be pondered for longer than just 1/24th of a second. Or maybe it's because I just always liked comic books.

It is extremely pleasant to touch pen and ink or graphite to paper in forming what I imagine or have actually seen. Give me some nice paper, pencils, and pens and I am happy. For me, the magic of creating a drawing is the same as the magic of exposing an image on film.

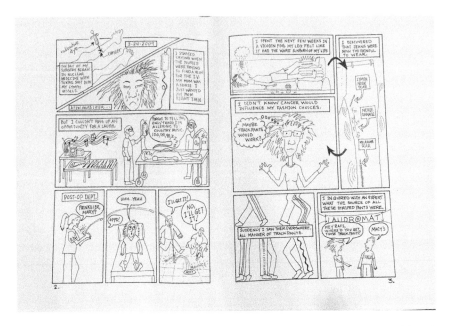

Figure 8.6 Mary E. Walter: "Cancer-Y Enough: A Heartwarming Story of Grief, Cancer and Track Pants Mini-Comic-Books," Sakura micron ink on Bristol paper, 2010, p. 2, 3.

I create stories drawn from my own experiences and encounters in the wider world, the comedy and tragedy of everyday life or just feelings or emotions that have been seared into my heart or psychological storage bank. I want to reduce the images I create into the simplest forms possible to make a cartoon or advertising-like impact.

I am fascinated with the expression of contrast, whether that between dark and light, chiaroscuro, colors, shapes, edges or what people say and what people actually do. I also love to depict the nature of various cultures, whether that be a very small grouping of people or that of a country that I have visited. Creating art and storytelling have been deeply therapeutic for me during this difficult time of healing from cancer and all other traumata that followed my diagnosis surgery (Figure 8.6).

5   **"CANCER-Y ENOUGH"** *page 2 & 3,* Mary E. Walter, 2010, double-page spread, mini-comic book published size: 5 1/2" × 8 1/2", photocopy on paper (original art: two side by side 9" × 12" pages, Sakura micron ink pen on Bristol paper).

The day of my surgery was surreal. I had no idea how profoundly my life would change in one day. Only afterwards, in a Vicodin fog, could I reflect

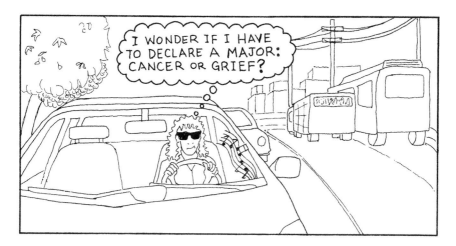

Figure 8.7 Mary E. Walter: "Double Major, Front Cover," Sakura micro ink on Bristol paper.

on the lightning speed of the 12 days between diagnosis and tears, fear, grief, anxiety, depression and my discovery of track pants as a solution to the pain in my leg (Figure 8.7).

6   *"DOUBLE MAJOR" front cover, Mary E. Walter, 2011, mini-comic book published size: 5 1/2" × 8 1/2", photocopy on paper (original art: 9" × 12", Sakura Micron ink pen on Bristol paper).*

In Los Angeles, where I live, we spend a lot of time in our cars, alone, driving to and fro with our thoughts to keep us company. I would often wonder during this time, when I saw another driver violate some rule of the road, if they were also finding it difficult to concentrate, maybe trying to decide which major to declare. I was so spaced out and in shock I shouldn't have been driving. I found out later that an inability to concentrate is one of the symptoms of a cancer diagnosis, as well as grieving and PTSD, all of which I was experiencing (Figure 8.8).

7   *"DOUBLE MAJOR" page 7, Mary E. Walter, 2011, mini-comic book published size: 5 1/2" × 8 1/2", photocopy on paper (original art: 9" × 12" page, Sakura micron ink pen on Bristol paper).*

I have travelled to many foreign cultures in my life. I didn't expect to be encountering two new cultures I had never seen before: the cancer world and the grieving world. The cancer community had a lot of death happening. The grieving community was the aftermath of the other, what is left behind.

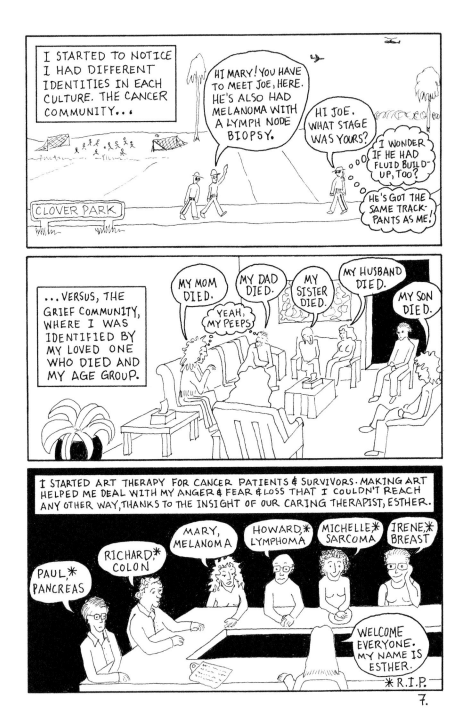

Figure 8.8 Mary E. Walter: "Double Major," Sakura micro ink on Bristol paper, p. 7.

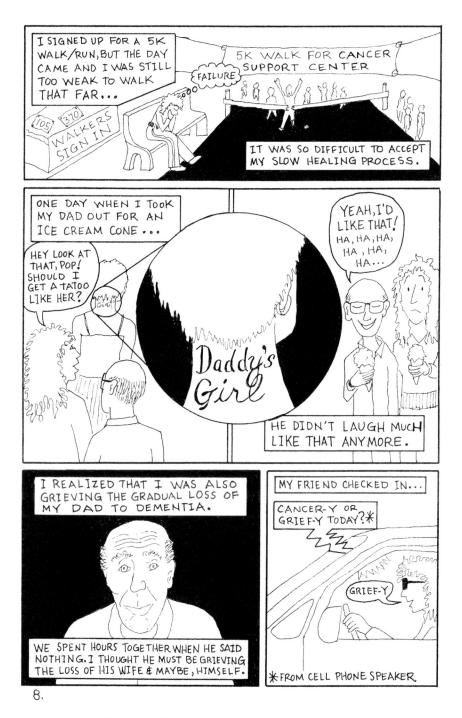

8.

Figure 8.9 Mary E. Walter: "Double Major," Sakura micro ink on Bristol paper, p. 8.

I had to be careful not to bring one world into the other. People from both cultures weren't comfortable hearing that I lived in both worlds. I grew to love those I sat next to each week, who I could share from my soul, without judgment from them, the horrors from each world (Figure 8.9).

8   *"DOUBLE MAJOR" page 8, Mary E. Walter, 2011, mini-comic book published size: 5 1/2" × 8 1/2", photocopy on paper (original art: 9" × 12" page, Sakura micron ink pen on Bristol paper).*

I was so disappointed in how slowly my body was healing. I was also grieving the gradual loss of my father. There were the fleeting joyful and surprising moments I spent with my Dad, who was in decline from dementia. He would spark to life and fade away. He was going away. I was hardly there myself (Figure 8.10).

9   *"FROM TRACK PANTS TO YOGA PANTS" page 6, Mary E. Walter, 2011, mini-comic book published size: 5 1/2" × 8 1/2", photocopy on paper (original art: 4" × 7" panel from 9" × 12" page, Sakura micron ink pen on Bristol paper).*

Life doesn't stop because of cancer and grieving. I took to yoga with a vengeance and exhausted myself. The multiple and minute instructions of yoga helped tremendously with concentration. My father was also grieving the loss of his wife (my mother) of 58 years. I tried to remind myself to have gratitude and tenderness in all things: my yoga, my Dad and myself (Figure 8.11).

10   *"FROM TRACK PANTS TO YOGA PANTS" page 9, Mary E. Walter, 2011, top panel only, mini-comic book published size: 5 1/2" × 8 1/2", photocopy on paper (original art: 4" × 7" panel from 9" × 12" page, Sakura micron ink pen on Bristol paper).*

My friends from the cancer support group who also had melanoma became my "gang" who I could depend on for all kinds of current information about this form of cancer, who knew which doctors were good and which were bad, who knew treatment options, and who generally just kicked my butt in pointing out how lucky I was to have stage one. I loved them for their bravery in the face of death and for caring enough to tell me the truth.

Some thoughts

Esther Dreifuss-Kattan

Mary Walter, with her many artistic talents, used her new skills as a comic book writer and illustrator to work through her multiple traumata and personal losses at the time of her cancer. Thinking in defined picture boxes

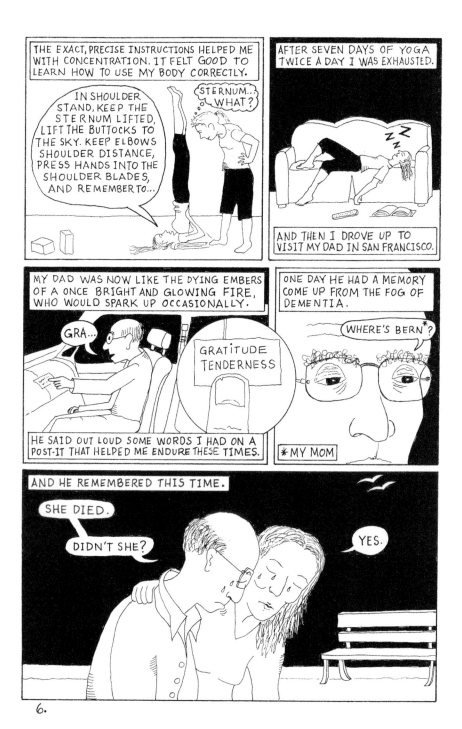

6.

Figure 8.10 Mary E Walter: "From Track Pants to Yoga Pants," p. 6.

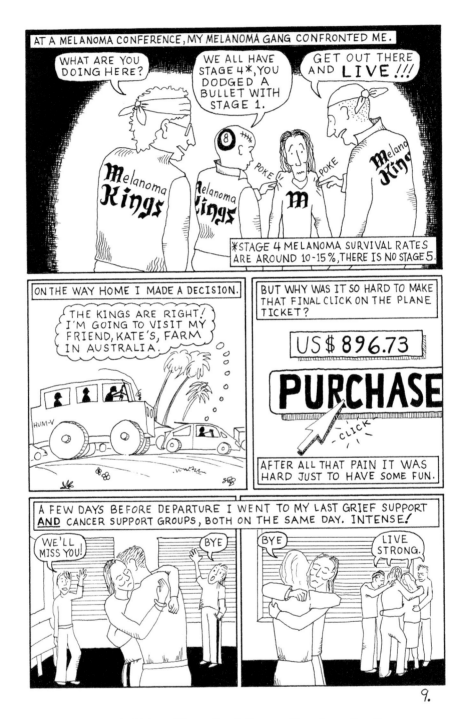

Figure 8.11 Mary E Walter: "From Track Pant to Yoga Pants," p. 9.

provided a sense of order in representing the world of facts, and her creative concentration offered armor against psychological and physical pain. Marking her new reality and new or recovered emotions with a new form allowed for a new sense of union with her different group members. Mary very skillfully crafted each panel, using her "imaginative muscles" (Wilner, 1977, p. 144) and thus aided in her slow recovery. Her focused creative concentration and exploration of her cancer journey, combined with mourning important losses—like her mother, an impaired leg, and eventually her father, with their related emotional impacts—achieved a union not only between her conscious and unconscious world, but also with her friends in the different cancer support groups and in her comic book class. Putting feelings such as anger, fears, confusion and mourning into her comic book design, while tracing her bodily experiences and showcasing movement with words, helped in the renewed integration of mind and body, addressing the self in relation to the other. Because of her precise remembering through drawing, she achieved an inner power of perception and new insight into her own psyche. In an attempt to take some distance from it by externalizing it into her comic books, Mary was prepared through art making to revisit and confront with her conscious creative inner eye both her cancer with its pain, and her family loss,. Her imaginative abilities helped this artist to stand again on a more solid ground, not only with both legs but with new psychic and artistic resources, using lines to create her forms, embracing her new physical and psychological geography. These comic books of Mary's journey with melanoma and loss restored her sense of self and strengthened the artists' inner balance, in an attempt to restore in the outside what was lost from the inside, namely a sense of security.

Creating colorful forms and symbols in her collages and cutouts had helped Mary in the working-through process of her multiple trauma in real time, while the speech bubbles in her comic strips, with their sometimes fun dialogues, dealt more with the group process and finding her personal place in it. Mary addressed overwhelming experiences with her family and the medical staff and later expanded in her comic books on her continuing journey to a successful cure from melanoma and its side effects. In the comic books, Mary also addressed her survival guilt, as she had a curable stage 1 of melanoma, unlike other patients and friends in the Cancer and Creativity group, and in other groups that contemplate death from melanoma. Unfortunately some members in these groups died while Mary was a participant. These losses not only bought forth sadness and mourning but revived her survivor guilt.

While Mary was able to transform her cancer trauma initially with the help of cutouts and collages, she was later able to elaborate them into reflections through comic book panels that initially were depressing and upsetting, but later became humorous. The panels of the comic books offered secure frames where she could outline and contain scene after scene, one problem or insight after the other, as she had experienced it in her real journey with melanoma. It offered her a creative and contained space to memorialize not only the challenging time fighting cancer but also the important people in her life, both alive and now dead, and thus achieving a sense of wholeness and reparation. While the paper cut-out collages addressed more specific challenging situations with oncologists and family issues before and during Mary's journey with cancer, the comic book panels made light of her more social journey with cancer and with several cancer support groups. Both were very helpful for Mary who is used to thinking in picture frames, being a true artist in her field as a visual effects editor in Hollywood. Being in a comic book class with mostly younger and healthy participants helped Mary get perspective on her own cancer journey and to recover her sense of humor. Slowly after the relief when her Melanoma was eliminated by surgery on her leg, Mary realized that she saw herself as a healthy person again.

References

Wilner, M. (1977). Foreword by Anna Freud. *On Not Being Able to Paint*. An H-B-B Paperback. London: Heinemann.

Chapter 9

Cancer maps and superheroes

Children and adolescents express their cancer journey

Esther Dreifuss-Kattan

Artists: several kids

Introduction

My interest in art therapy with children is inspired by my late mentor and later dissertation advisor Edith Kramer, a practicing artist, one of the founders of art therapy with children, and the first professor at the NYU Art Therapy program. Kramer was psychoanalyzed in the 1930s by Annie Reich, a well-known psychoanalyst in Vienna. Kramer wrote many books on art therapy with children and teenagers over the course of her long life, starting in 1959. Kramer's books, informed by her knowledge of psychoanalytic concepts and by her own clinical experience were the first on the subject of art therapy I read and introduced me to the field.

When Kramer was 17, during her final exams at her gymnasium secondary school, her mother gave her Freud's *Introductory Lectures on Psychoanalysis*, which marked the very beginning of her interest in Freud. She described how fortunate she was to have grown up in Vienna, close to Freudian psychoanalysis and to the progressive art education movement led by Victor Loewenfeld, who worked with the blind (Loewenfeld, 1947). The city was the European center of culture, a "bohemian environment full of actors, psychoanalysts, artists, and revolutionaries" (Kramer, 2017, p. xvi).

She also recalled how she could see Anna and Sigmund Freud strolling around the lake at Grundlsee, the beautiful Austrian mountain town where her family maintained a vacation resort (Dreifuss-Kattan, 1983). Psychoanalysts Wilhelm and Annie Reich, Hans Sachs and Otto Fenichel also used to vacation there with their families, as did well-known Viennese writers and poets.

When Edith was 12 years old she started to take art classes in Vienna with Friedl Dicker, a family friend, Friedl, a practicing artist, was a student of Johannes Itten who left Vienna to teach at the Bauhaus. Edith Kramer moved later with Friedl to Prague, when Vienna became too dangerous for resident Jews. Edith describes her relationship with Dicker as an apprenticeship between student and master, though both started psychoanalysis with

Annie Reich during their time together. Together they taught art to immigrant children who had fled Nazi Germany, leading to the first time Kramer saw the chaotic imagery of pictures by children who had been traumatized and uprooted. She was saddened to realize from distorted body images that they identified with the aggressor (Makarove, 2017, p. 39).

Kramer managed to catch the last boat leaving from Poland to New York in 1938, but Dicker was incarcerated in the Terezin concentration camp in 1942. Dicker continue to paint and give lessons to the children that were at Terezin, a model concentration camp intended to exhibit the ethical treatment of Jewish intellectuals, scientists and artists along with their families, before they were all deported to Auschwitz. Dicker made sure that all these children's pictures were dated and preserved (Kramer, 2017), in a collection that today is shown around the world. When its images appeared in Los Angeles in an exhibit honoring Friedl Dicker, Kramer was invited to speak about her late teacher. She and I saw these drawings together and she remarked how coherent the drawings made by internees were when compared with those by refugee children, and how the same traumas did not manifest in them. Kramer believed that Dicker must have integrated some of her knowledge of child development as well as used psychoanalytic insights to treat her art students. She also remembered that these children were in Terezin together with their parents, though sleeping separately in children's houses. Kramer concluded that the images' relative peacefulness testified to how the adults could protect these children from the daily murders and upheaval, and to the value of the holistic interplay between art teacher, or art therapist, and family in times of immense pain.

These conclusions were augmented when Kramer started to work in New York City. She treated traumatized and abandoned children and teenagers in the integrated Wiltwyck School for Boys in New York City, where she worked until 1947. Kramer's methods of art therapy went on to rely on providing her patients with quality art supplies, a safe and sheltering art studio and, importantly, a comfortable structure and a positive emotional environment. The most important piece of this environment was sufficient time: time allowed these kids and teenagers to experiment and create their art pieces without duress. I witnessed the care with which she implemented these principles for 30 years as an artist and teacher. She believed that when these elements combine successfully, real artistic expression conducive to a truthful therapeutic encounter could take place.

Art therapy for children with cancer

In this chapter I will address the benefits of art therapy groups, art-based creative programs and individual art therapy sessions for children, teenagers and young adults in different stages of cancer. These therapeutic encounters reflect methodologies that Edith Kramer pioneered and are indebted to her early work in treating traumatized children. I will focus on the physical and psychological concerns affecting children and teenagers with cancer, who must go through long, intensive and sometimes traumatic treatments, and their accompanying feelings of anxiety, depression, social isolation and even post-traumatic stress disorder. To explain the art therapy process and the psychosocial significance of the creative connection that develops over its course between art therapists and the children impacted by serious illness, I would like to start with a dialogue from the famous story The *Little Prince*, written by the French writer Antoine de Saint-Exupery, and first published in 1943 during the Second World War. Here, a pilot who is stranded in the desert converses with a little prince he has encountered while waiting for help. The little prince asks the pilot to draw him a little sheep:

> "This is only his box. The sheep you asked for is inside," says the pilot to the discontent little prince, who wanted him to draw a sheep.
>
> I was very surprised to see a light break over the face of my young judge:
>
> "That is exactly the way I wanted it! Do you think that this sheep will have to have a great deal of grass?"
>
> "Why?"
>
> "Because where I live everything is very small..."
>
> "There will surely be enough grass for him," I said. "It is a very small sheep that I have given you."
>
> He bent his head over the drawing:
>
> "Not so small that—Look! He has gone to sleep..."
>
> And that is how I made the acquaintance of the little prince.
>
> (De Saint-Exupery, 1943)

In this short dialogue between the pilot and the little prince, the author demonstrates how children of all ages love to lead us through their imaginative stories and decode their internal imagery, if we are open to being guided along. The little prince just needs the drawing of a little box to become acquainted with his little imaginary sheep inside the box. This box, or really this piece of paper (or a canvas in art therapy) provides a safe space for imagination and creativity to flourish at a time of fear, isolation or medical trauma, a time signified in Saint-Exupery's story by the war understood to surround his characters. With the help of the supportive pilot companion, the child's fantasy life can grow, as the grass does for the sheep. Then, our little prince—like all children, healthy or sick, sad or happy—are ready to take us to imagined distant planets, including the unconscious one.

An analogous process takes place in art therapy. In the art therapy group we stage a meeting between the inner world of the sick children, impacted by serious illness and the external reality represented by the art therapists, mediated by the creative environment of an art space with colors, papers, fabric, strings, clay and wood. The picture, painting or sculpture precisely occupies the area between inner world and reality, the transitional space that allows the painting or sculpture to become a transitional object, a bridge between the inner and outer worlds of the participants that are both separated yet interrelated.

Long before she develops the capacity for language, the infant becomes aware of her own new world through sensory events, later abstracted and formulated into images. Even after we become able to communicate, many of our internal states are very deep, very private and beyond the reach of words. Children's internal or unconscious worlds often remain inaccessible through verbal communication, but can be easily expressed and observed in imaginary play, scribbles, drawing or painting or any other creative expression. As the pilot offered an empty box that left plenty of space for the little prince's dream to emerge from the unconscious, the art therapist offers an idea or merely a physical presence that allows the young patient with cancer to see potential truths about himself or herself through creative play.

As we read earlier, the English pediatrician and psychoanalyst D. W. Winnicott expostulated that the transitional object, transitional space and the various transitional phenomena that succeed it form the foundation for all creative activity. As such transitional phenomena, the canvas or piece of paper can become a creative stage and the paint or clay can become a great medium, as well as a favorite activity for children and adolescents with cancer, warding off extreme fears and anxieties; art is a vehicle to transform these emotional states creatively and register fantasies, hopes, inner conflicts and expectations.

As imaginary play results in a concrete form through colors and brush, fabric or paper and scissors, engendering miraculous art pieces, psychological insights become interpretable within the safe space of the patient's relationship with his art therapist. Art therapy can result eventually in a renewed psychological balance, stabilizing the young cancer patient's self. Through this relationship, and the creative working-through process, the art piece can have a lasting physical legacy and also connect patients to their peers in the group or to their families.

Pediatric cancer

Only 1% of all new cancer patients in the United States are younger than 20 years old. Of these, 40% are diagnosed with leukemia in its various forms, such as lymphoblastic leukemia (ALL), acute myeloid leukemia (AML), or lymphomas. Other common pediatric cancers include brain tumors such as astrocytoma, brain and spinal cord tumors, brainstem glioma, neuroplastoma solid tumors such as Wilms tumor or Ewing sarcomas. While children between the ages of two and nine have a 70% chance to survive a diagnosis of ALL leukemia, cancer is often not easily diagnosed, sharing symptoms with regular infections and flu-like fatigue, bone pains and fever. A leukemia diagnosis thus might take several weeks or even months and visits to different doctors to achieve a diagnosis. Children from infancy to teenage years diagnosed with leukemia or lymphoma have to go through grueling, long-term ambulatory therapy and chemotherapy regimes, followed or sometimes ending with radiation therapy. For some leukemia patients, after the more acute chemotherapy treatment is finished, it is followed by maintenance chemotherapy for two years. While this is less taxing and less toxic for the child, it must be balanced against the demands of their being back in school. If these treatments do not bring a full remission, bone marrow or stem cell transplantation may be required, which necessitate longer hospitalizations and bring forth more severe physical as well as psychological side effects. While life-saving, these extreme treatments demand long-term rehabilitation, both psychologically as well as physically. The same is true for solid tumors and Ewing's sarcoma, which are often treated first with surgeries and radiation and/or chemotherapy treatments, followed by physical rehabilitation.

These long-term intrusive treatments can provoke major psychological reactions in the child with cancer and in their family. They become obsessed with the child's survival, and with preventing infections that could potentially be lethal because of the child's compromised immune system. Since every infection, even a moderate fever, can result in hospitalization and separation, massive costs for treatment can aggravate a family's constant worry over health risks, and can add to these stressors to precipitate post-traumatic stress disorders, depression and acute separation anxiety, the latter especially in smaller children with cancer.

One of the primary goals of art therapy is to bring forth and understand the internal world of our young cancer patients. We strive to make their inner world visible and accessible for exploration, search for the meanings to ameliorate physical and psychological pain, and foster psychological growth, insight and joy in spite of cancer and its often-long term, intense treatments. If we are to communicate effectively with our sometimes very young patients it is essential to discover a common language. In order to avoid being stuck alone in the desert like our little prince, the young patient in the bed in a hospital or outpatient clinic, we can make use of their imagination and creativity to gain psychological insights.

In the process of fighting a potential life-threatening and/or chronic illness, the child or teenager's self-worth is continually threatened by intrusive treatments that can result in anxieties, depression, fears and trauma. Long treatments or chronic pain can destroy the child's ability to play, meet with peers and be an active member of his or her family. This loss can cause sadness and a sense of isolation, burgeoning into the source of deep psychological pain. Moreover teenagers may realize what a burden their illness and treatment might be on parents' professional and private lives, leading to guilt or resentment. This can be particularly acute when they overhear fights about responsibility for care, or who has to take them to the hospital or doctor visits. Not that care is actually easy: parents may very well need support from their extended family, the community and from their friends so they can take a day off to catch up on sleep, or see a therapist themselves. Psychological or art therapeutic care allows children to voice concerns, explicitly or unconsciously, rather than internalizing them. Reparative processes such as art therapy help to reestablish the integrity of the self against this essential-seeming difference the child may feel from others. It can give rise to creative transformation that can establish a new and different personal narrative (Councill, 1993).

I remember working with a freshman in high school, Nina, who was diagnosed with Ewing Sarcoma behind her shoulder. The tumor needed to be removed surgically, wherein doctors would replace the infected bone with an iron plate. Long hospitalizations for chemo, two younger siblings and an unstable marriage between her parents led to plenty of tensions within the family, all contributing to Nina feeling confused and depressed. She did not want to see her friends or for them to see her, though there was some contact by phone. I tried to find out what she wanted to do when she grew up and she told me she wanted to be a singer, since she loved music.

I suggested that she paint a picture about music. It took her several sessions to complete the canvas, in her precise, artistic manner. With her consent, I also invited, her parents to discuss (without Nina present) how they could lower the tension at home. After Nina's picture finished, she was so happy and played for me the music she loved from her phone. I was duly impressed indeed. This teenage patient became more confident and focused less on her cancer and more beautiful pictures followed, at a time when she could not yet focus on her school work. After over a year of treatment she went back to school, concentrated on her academics and graduated from high school. Now in college, Nina would like to become a psychologist. At the time of Nina's total isolation and insecurity, caused by physical loss and social isolation as well as by the fear of death that was her daily reality, we found the one thing, music, that made her happy and helped her become more self-confident. Art making transformed this teenager, in conjunction with her parents' collaboration. Most importantly was the insistence of Nina's mother on locating the most qualified surgeon in town to perform the challenging bone removal. Together, these interventions helped Nina to survive physically and psychologically, and to become a self-confident young adult with an interesting social circle.

Artistic expression and play for kids and teenagers with cancer can be a call for respite or a wish for some control in an otherwise uncontrollable environment. Some young patients develop a strong need to work creatively throughout their affliction with cancer, using art, photography, video, social media or email narratives in order to keep their psychosocial environment with peers and parents intact and to attempt to make sense of their psychological and physical impediments, and their feelings of depression due to their illness and its treatments.

Severe illness transforms the landscape and routines of these children's lives. Children of all ages impacted by cancer are confronted with short- and long-term hospitalizations to recover from surgery, extreme side-effects of medication, low immune systems or low white blood cell counts that makes them very vulnerable for infection and for pain control or palliative care. Leukemia patients and others are repeatedly stuck with needles to check their blood cell count and undergo chemotherapy that makes their hair fall out and leaves them very tired and irritable. A port is usually surgically inserted under their skin for easy access to their vein for chemotherapy; the insertion can be a traumatic procedure, with the port itself looking aesthetically unpleasant and needing regular flushing by health workers to prevent infection. Children with cancer need to be careful with their physical activities so they do not get injured, nor infected by their friend's cold, or by the school's door handle. Frequent visits to the ER are common at all hours of the day or night.

The trauma experienced by children and parents as a result of this re-structuring of their lives is significant. Some children become compliant and quiet, turning into imitations of 'good' children. Hugger compares them to abused children (Hugger, 2005, p. 412). Fears can also overwhelm a small child, or even a near adult, when he or she has to take several pills at one specific time several times a week, or has to be restrained because of a shot or procedure. In the latter case, whoever is the main supporter of the child's medical care must also take on the role of a supportive ego for the sick child. Then, the patient will be able to relax more in the face of a re-traumatization by the medical procedure. A young adult patient I was treating was very thankful when I suggested to his parents that his father should take over an informal supervision of the patient's ambulatory chemotherapy each week, in order to help him begin sleeping again, relax, and reduce his high state of anxiety. His father's presence and focused watch there achieved precisely this effect.

Some mothers or fathers with a severely sick child break down when their child is confronted with severe medical intervention, such as a biopsy, general anesthesia or reoccurrence of illness, especially when the child is very young, and feels overwhelmed or even traumatized by medical interventions and inundated by overwhelming fears. While adults have more of the ability to block out overwhelming emotions when needed, children have much less and easily become flooded by them, resulting in dissociation or inducing trauma that can trigger empathetic catastrophes in their parents. Attempts to protect children from infection can also lead to social isolation from friends and close family members, such as siblings, cousins and aunts, uncles or teachers. Teenagers are often particularly impacted by social isolation, missing their peers and an active social life more acutely because they just gained more independence from home and family. For older kids and teenagers, social media such as Facebook, Skype interaction, texting and artistic expression of any kind, like photography, art, music, drawing comic books, writing and illustrating, knitting and composing are of great benefit, since both, in different ways, can reduce isolation. When teenagers and other child patients communicate their physical setbacks or losses with peers through social media, their frustration, anger and fears diminish. They engender support and cheer up, and fortify their friendships without the fear of infections.

One example of such communication among child patients is the "Color My World" program designed by two art therapists, Alyssa Wiesel and I, with the help of Randi Grossman, the executive director of the not-for-profit organization Chai Lifeline, formed to help families who have a child, teenager or young adult with cancer. I will address how art therapy and art based programs like "Color My World" can help work through psychological issues faced by pediatric cancer patients and their siblings. "Color My World" invites children and teenagers of all ages that have cancer or are cancer survivors to meet together. These smaller groups, exclusively for pediatric cancer patients and survivors of different ages, foster personal interaction through the sharing of similar (or very different) personal medical histories of their illness, using creativity and artistic expression. When leading these groups, we introduce a specific theme that we share with the participants, and particular media or materials to go with the theme, before a given group event. These two-hour long groups result in a genuine artistic expression, insightful engagement with each other's painting or drawing and discussion between patients of different ages and the art therapists, animating an open, playful, and supportive group setting.

In one group we asked each participant to create their personal cancer map, basically an illustration of their experience with cancer as a journey. I have excerpted some descriptions by the art therapy patients of their pieces below (Figure 9.1):

Map by Jeff, a "cancer warrior" age 13, writes:

> At the beginning I was confused; I did not know what happened. That is why I made the road twist, and I made a "Q" [glued on a Q Scrabble piece] to represent the 'Question' I had. Then the road is straight with needles to represent the entire hospital visit. Finally, I put the airplane shooting a scary animal to show the end of my treatment, when my medicine [chemotherapy] killed the cancer.

Jeff lets us know how confusing it was for him, until he could be properly diagnosed and understood that his cancer could be treated. The hospital visits he represents with needles, an overall painful experience symbolized with pricking for blood samples and receiving chemotherapy. A small plastic animal represented the cancer, an alive creature like a cancer cell that looks grim and needed to be killed for Jeff to live (Figure 9.2).

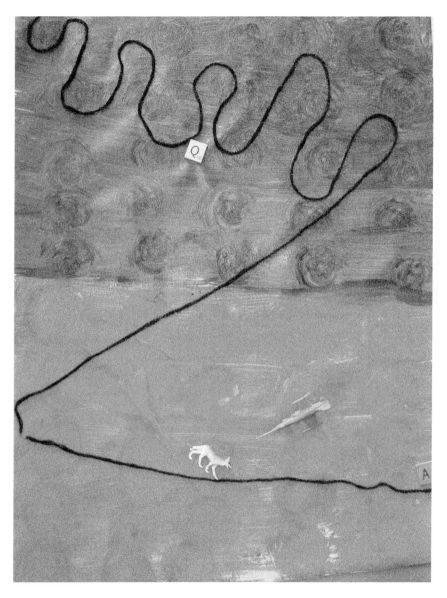

Figure 9.1 Jeff, "My Cancer Map," Acrylic, Plastic Fire, Wool, Scrabble Piece, 2013.

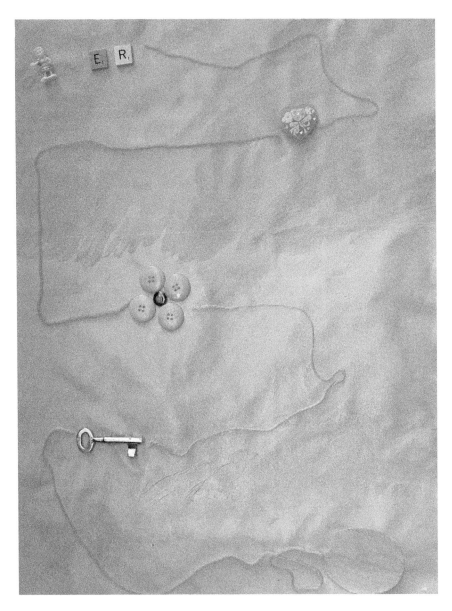

Figure 9.2 Chaya Spatler, "My Cancer Map," Acrylic Paint, Wool, Buttons, Plastic Figure, Metal Key.

Chaya, "cancer warrior" age 9 writes:

> The person on the canvas trapped in a string is me in the emergency room, when I did not understand anything the doctors and nurses were doing or saying. Then they figured out that I had Ewing sarcoma, so everyone started feeling bad and gave me attention and presents, represented by the heart. Then the string is straight because it was calm in my life since I realized what was happening. The flower shows that like a flower needs sunshine to get strong, I needed chemotherapy to get better. The key represents opening the lock to feeling better as I got to the end of my chemotherapy. The yellow circle shines bright to show that I am better now and can do all the fun things I want.

While Chaya describes a similar scene, it has a very different tone. It seems that this little girl could relax more once she actually felt her cancer had a name and the doctors knew how to treat it. She also emphasizes how love and care together with attention and presents helped her to relax more and go with the flow of the chemo protocol and hospital visits. Both of these children were very happy to play with all the fun art materials in the "Color My World" sessions and each was able to reflect uniquely on what might seem like a common event.

Another creative group concept we offer is a "Paintbrush Partners" program. Healthy volunteer high school students partner with a child or teenager with cancer, a sibling of a cancer patient, or with a survivor. Together, they collaborate on a painting, collage or sculpture, depicting an everyday topic they arrive at in common like their favorite superhero, their favorite place to hang out when being alone, or other themes that might relate more to their medical circumstances. Art therapists issue these themes at each particular workshop. Paintbrush Partners without cancer are trained and selected because they are open, kind and accepting of the sick children, taught to see them as whole persons despite their illnesses and personal losses. Paintbrush Partners help their sick children or their siblings to connect with their playful, inner creative well. We instruct them not to ask intrusive questions but rather to listen empathically to their younger friends and respond to questions elucidating the art project if it is not understood. These Paintbrush Partners also assist their partners in technique, helping them to choose colors, clean their brushes and execute their pieces practically, without influencing or telling them what to paint or how to paint it. The younger artists are permitted to come up with their own genuine and meaningful personal imagery.

The art therapeutic assistance that Paintbrush Partners offers is aptly summed up by the concept of the "third hand," one of Edith Kramer's theories: "a hand that helps the creative process along without being intrusive, without distorting meaning or imposing pictorial ideas or preferences alien to the client" (Kramer & Gerity, 2000, p. 48). The third hand of the Paintbrush Partner helps younger kids to get over their shyness; it encourages their artistic expression while they gain a new friend who is not much older, and they relax so they can work artistically in a bigger group where they may not necessarily know all the other members.

These artistic, supportive partnerships between younger cancer patients and older peers last a couple of hours per session, and are guided and observed by the attending two art therapists. The younger cancer patients love to partner up with older kids and often form close, lasting relationships with them, that are not only reflected in the wonderful paintings, collages and portraits, but are mirrored in the eyes and smiles of the child artists who love to create art together with older partners whom they admire. Art making is a restorative, healing process, and the painting or collage becomes a subject of pride, or can become a personal gift that can be shared with parents or other sick children and teenagers. After the art piece is completed, the Paintbrush Partner and art therapist assist the artists to share their thoughts about their creation and help them to write it up in descriptions like the above. Each group session, and sharing of work, is always followed by clapping and cheering.

The teenage volunteer, on the other hand develops empathy and compassion while observing what it means to have cancer and in what way kids can be affected by it. They learn, often to their surprise, that in spite of cancer these younger and older sick children have the same ambitions, focus and perseverance as other children without cancer. They enjoy being role models and often recognize that their own creative needs are not met, due to school pressure or other reasons, and ask to do their own art projects. Both the volunteers and the cancer survivors often choose service or palliative professions when they are old enough to go to college and graduate schools.

As we see in Chaya's and Jeff's cancer maps, children are confused by their sudden illness; art-therapeutic mentorships are valuable precisely as creative guidance, as children must develop their own ways to make sense of the new and overwhelming world into which they are thrown. Many new adults confront these children in a very private way, in the unfamiliar environment of the big hospital complex and the very active, confusing outpatient clinic. They get pricked, their bodies are touched and examined by many doctors and nurses and scanned by huge and powerful machines, and they have to swallow or have infusions of unpleasant, strong-tasting cancer drugs that make them very sick or alter their behavior and mental states. There exists no prescribed, clear recipe for dealing with cancer, hence the need for creative invention.

Invention, however, can be misinformed. These children wonder why they got cancer, and what might reason it might possibly have. Some believe that they are being punished because of angry thoughts they harbored towards a sibling or parent. Others believe their bad behavior or school problems are the cause, or their dependency on a parent might result in weakness and illness. Often, at the first consultation with the pediatric oncologist, the doctor explains to the family and to the child or teenager with cancer that nobody know why these illnesses appear, although he or she will stress that they are not karmic or punitive in the way children might imagine. Although this stipulation can alleviate some fears, sometimes it does not really help.

That is why art therapy and play therapy/psychotherapy for children with cancer are so very essential (Hugger, 2005). Art therapy/psychotherapy can address these confusing thoughts and fears, and the misplaced guilt or sense of responsibility that often are communicated in children's drawings, doodles or paintings, and address the psychic numbing that repeated exposure to them may cause, or which may arise as a misguided defense against them.

In addition to a child's misperception that he or she is responsible for cancer, chemotherapy, newer immune therapies, radiation and surgeries can all assault the child's body and can change his or her body image, resulting in embarrassment and low self-esteem that can lead to social withdrawal. A diminished sense of self-worth can lead to sleeping a lot or not wanting to venture out, or to losing interest in seeing friends, siblings or relatives. These behaviors can be symptoms of depression or of separation anxiety. They also can indicate that, while grieving for or processing their diagnosis, the young patient is not yet ready to be sociable, or that he or she is just too physically ill (Figure 9.3).

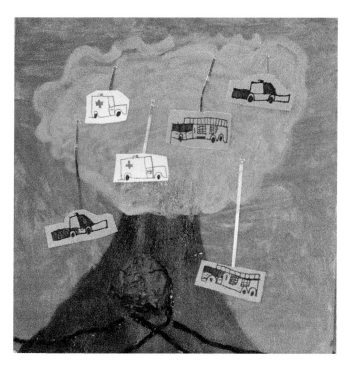

Figure 9.3 Adam Pomeranz, "Tree of Life-My Rescue Tree," Acrylic Paint, Paper, Magic Marker.

Tree of Life: acrylic paint with paper collage on string:
Adam, "cancer warrior," age 7; Aviv, "Paintbrush Partner," age 16

Adam was battling leukemia for over a year by the time he made this picture together with his Paintbrush Partner, Aviv. The theme given to them was to create a Tree of Life. Together, they painted the tree with green and brown acrylic paint on a green background, this juxtaposition indicating perhaps that there might be other trees, or grass for the tree to grow from and thrive. The trunk is strong and large enough to hold up a large canopy and the roots extend far downward, represented by brown paint and by brown strings. In the place of fruits, leaves, or nesting birds, Adam's tree shelters two ambulances and two fire trucks in its branches. These are sketched on separate pieces of red and white paper with markers, and hung on the tree with long strips of red masking tape.

Adam imagines here the ambulance he might need in case of emergency to get to the hospital in time. Like all little boys, he loves fire trucks, but for a young leukemia patient they might represent the protection of professionals who could assuage the ravages of cancer inside him, as well as dampen the rages that arise as the side effects of the steroids Adam has to take in addition to his chemotherapy. Instead of living the life of a regular boy who loves sports and can play with peers in school, Adam is confronted with mood changes, multiple fears, and confusing treatments, and is often cannot go to school because he is too sick, or to prevent infections. Despite his misfortune, Adam fought like a "cancer warrior" and comported himself like a hero in the hospital and in the outpatient clinic where his nurses and doctors loved him. He also felt at ease with his warm and compassionate family (Figure 9.4).

A year later, at age 8, Adam was asked together with his paintbrush partner Harris to make a self-portrait with acrylic paint on canvas. The portrait was not required to be realistic or "accurate" in a conventional sense; Adam sees himself in this painting as an Israeli general in uniform with a tough, but also funny, face. As an immigrant from Israel, Adam still identifies with his birth country. Chemotherapy and sporadic overnight hospitalizations are a challenge that Adam and his family had already endured, at this point, for two years. Adam wishes unconsciously, in this portrait, to hide his anguish and frustration behind the toughness and bravery of a military leader capable of defeating cancer, while maintaining a sense of humor and nonchalance even in adversity. Adam, incidentally, did just that and is a healthy teenager now (Figure 9.5).

Picture 5: Self-Portrait: Super Hero
Ari "cancer warrior," age 4, with Aviv, "Paintbrush Partner," age 16

Ari went through three years of rigorous chemotherapy regimes. Asked to create the same type of fictionalized self-portrait as Adam, he immediately identified with Batman, his favorite superhero. He worked enthusiastically with his partner to create a black felt mask and cape. The wish

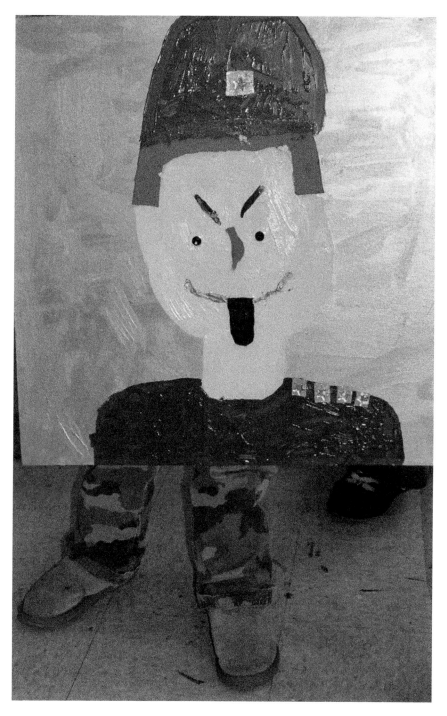

Figure 9.4 Adam Pomeranz, "Self Portrait-Superhero: Soldier," Acrylic Paint, Part of His Own Legs and Shoes.

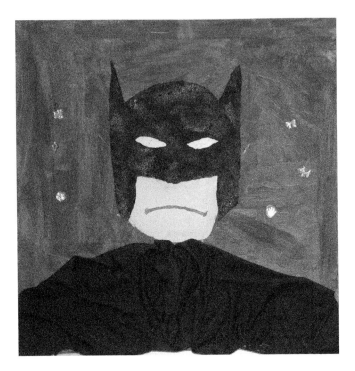

Figure 9.5 Ari, "Self-Portrait-Superhero: Batman," Acrylic Paint, Lack Felt, Glass Beads.

to be with the Batman illustrates his desire to become indestructible, a powerful superhero, strong enough to save all people, including himself, from an evil and destructive cancer. Aviel was so proud of this big canvas, for which he received so many compliments, and that strengthened his self-confidence immensely. Perhaps appropriately, collaging Batman allowed him for a while to forget his cancer by taking on a fantastic, heroic alter-ego, (as a talented, exceptional artist) that is exceptional.

With new relationship to the art-psychotherapist and the paintbrush partner, art therapy can help reestablish trust in others and sociability with the new relationship to the art therapist it constructs. Therapy reaffirms a stronger, new sense of self as an artist, while finding a comfortable state and place for play in the transitional space. Art therapy allows the sick or recovering child with cancer, a sense of mastery over their cancer experience, and the art studio becomes eventually a safe space away from the syringes and chemo drugs. The pediatric cancer patient's ability to choose and control his or her own colors, words and imagery without outside pressure or evaluation, can be particularly significant in building confidence and self-mastery, as the child's illness is being controlled all the time by parents, nurses, doctors, medications and often by a strict daily routine. Having regular art therapy appointments—whether in the hospital, the oncology outpatient clinic, or in private practice—can aid the child with any cancer in the process of adaptation to a new body image, after losing hair, a body part or function through chemotherapy, or internal or external surgery. Art psychotherapy helps reduce depression and decrease anxieties through nonverbal artistic expression. I have seen many times that it can also reduce pain by distraction, restore self-confidence and facilitate verbal communication, putting the feelings from the painting into words for the therapist and later for her family. Unconscious imagery will surface through art and play and thus becomes conscious and can be interpreted and help in the working-through process of loss, mourning and trauma. The close relationship between the therapist and a teenager or little child with cancer allows these more unconscious and conscious issues to be addressed, such as the loss of a body part or the fear and anger of having to live with chemotherapy for another two years. Some kids only like to have pictorial dialogues with the art therapist and not much talk, others like to play act them out, using the toys in my office in real time. I remember a little boy who took out the doctor suitcase play kit and wanted first to be my doctor and I was the patient and he roughed me up a bit and then it was followed by several sessions when he wanted to be the patient and he would tell me what I could to as the doctor. He mostly wanted tender love and care. That playacting allowed him to be finally in control and asked for all the attention love, and security he needed, outside of his family. Perhaps he was aware he could not ask for more attention at home, that his parent had other siblings to take care of and were stressed out.

Due to long term illness and its treatment, younger children and teenagers often regress, both physically, as well as psychologically, especially after surgery, intense chemotherapy and hospitalizations that can bring long term inactivity. Cancer treatments, hospital visits with their often intrusive and painful procedures like frequent blood-drawing, multiple symptoms and pain makes these young patients feel unbalanced and vulnerable. They become younger psychologically as well as physically than their stated age, dependent once again on their parents for walking, driving, lifting heavy objects, decision making, and discussion with health professionals, just when they thought they might have more freedom of movement and personal choices.

Once their body heals and their mind recovers from their potentially life-threatening experiences and they gain strength, these regressive patients become suddenly more mature then their healthy peers, having gone through grueling treatments, acute fears and near death experiences. Teenagers complain that they feel older than their classmates, recognizing their old friends as immature, and targeting childish behavior or social issues that the cancer survivors see as superficial and unimportant. Feeling younger in one period of their medical journey and prematurely aged after treatment can be very confusing for a child of any age, but particularly for teenagers, who face extra pressure to fit in, resent appearing different, and desire easy reintegration into school and social friendship circles.

Addressing subjects of guilt, poor self-image, and maturational displacement from peers in psychotherapy/art therapy, and sharing them with parents (if the teenage patient agrees), often helps resolve them. Other family members, such as cousins or older siblings, new friends who also went through cancer, or members of teenage cancer support groups, can also contributing to reducing patients' suffering from these issues, until the recovering child feels more psychologically stable, and better adapted. Once the young person recovers his or her self-confidence and physical integrity, they are ready to overcome their social isolation and can reach out to old friends.

Siblings of young and teenage cancer patients suffer from their own psychological issues. Their parents are focused emotionally and practically on their sick child, and have the unconscious tendency to neglect the psychological state of their healthy children, paradoxically in spite of parents' own intense worries, and the frequent doctor appointments, hospitalizations, financial insecurity that disrupt household routines. Siblings often express their psychological fears, or need for attention, through psychosomatic symptoms, such as headaches and stomachaches. They might refuse to go to school, a demand that may also originate in separation anxiety as parents frequently leave, and are often mentally distracted or absent despite being physically present. Siblings can become angry and resentful of being marginalized, leading to tantrums and trouble in school. Their own violence may also come from their sensitivity to anxious parents, parents poised to quarrel with each other over care for the sick child by tension and sleep deprivation. Smaller siblings may fear that cancer is contagious or that their behavior or even their fantasies helped to create the disease in their sibling. They might fear unconsciously that they will be punished, or that their parents are unable to protect them from illness, as they could not protect their sick sister or brother.

Art therapy with siblings of cancer patients is often a very successful and pleasurable education in working through these reactions. Expression through art can reduce siblings' anxiety, alleviate symptoms, and foster a connection to a secure object, like the art-psychotherapist at least once a week. Siblings may meet the therapist individually in the beginning, and later, when the family is more relaxed and the cancer patient is no longer in the active phase of treatment, could attend sessions with their entire family, as well as in an art group setting. This particular kind of "experiencing together" provides psychological support within the protected confines of the creative process and facilitates mutuality between the young cancer patients, their family, their friends in the group and the art therapist. Just as the transitional object in early childhood like a teddy bear or blanket can be used as a symbol for the absent mother during infancy, the drawing, painting, or created mask can become the mediating symbol of togetherness, persevering even through physical absence and associated suffering.

In one of the pictures, (not shown) nine-year-old Eva, the younger sister of a cancer patient, painted a Tree of Life that she called a "Candy Land Tree." The tree is a happy tree, a small child's dream tree. It only grows sweet things, from lollypops to M&M chocolate bits, to comfort Eva who is a little sad and lonely as her older sibling has cancer and parents are very busy and worry a lot. Both we adults as well as children use candy to comfort ourselves and a sibling of a cancer patient certainly has just cause. However, it's a strong tree, with a thick stable trunk with all the pink background, the favorite color of many small girls. Both color and content help this little girl to use this magic tree to have fun and relieve her anxiety and stress in this challenging time for her family.

Orly, the younger sister of a cancer patient, also aged nine, painted a similar tree of love, whose crown is a big green heart; the leaves on her tree are little hearts and the clouds are white hearts. Orly also needs a lot of love during an unstable time in her family because of her sibling's illness. Only extra love and attention from family and friends and/or from an art-psychotherapist still keeps this little sister psychologically stable and happy through this trying time. She craves love, as a little face, representing her most likely with a smile behind the tree looks out at us. Maybe saying, "Hello, I am here too, even though I am healthy."

It is the smile in this painting that brings forth how art is healing for this little sister. Not only could she paint with the help of her Paintbrush Partner and even use glitter glue to sign her name, she realized that it was acceptable to ask for comfort and be in the center of attention, proud as she was to have painted a big canvas. It's also fine to look for love and find it staring back at her from her picture. It is important for the parents to realize that there is enough love to go around for all children in the family in spite of illness.

References

Councill, T. (1993) Art Therapy with Pediatric Cancer Patients: Helping Normal Children Cope with Abnormal Circumstances. *Art Therapy: Journal of the American Art Therapy Association*, 10 (2), 78–87.

De Saint-Exupery, A. (1943) *2010 Worldsworth Classic*.

Dreifuss-Kattan (1982) Personal communication with Edith Kramer.

Gerity, L.A., & Anand, S. (Eds.) (2017) *The Legacy of Edith Kramer: A Multifaceted View*, Routledge, London and New York.

Hugger, L. (2005) The Psychological Treatment of Children Recovering from Leukemia. *Journal of Infant, Child, and Adolescent Psychotherapy*, 4 (4), 408–423.

Kramer, E. (2017) A Fortunate Life, Foreword. In: L.A. Gerity & S. Anand (Eds.)
The Legacy of Edith Kramer, Routledge, London and New York.

Kramer, E., & Gerity, L.A. (2000) *Art as Therapy. Collected paper*, Jessica Kingsley
Publishers, London.

Loewenfeld, V. (1947) *Creative and Mental Growth*, Macmillan, New York.

Macarova, E. (2017) Edith Kramer on Friedl Dicker-Brandeis, Erna Furman, and
Terezin: Interview with Elena Makarova. In: Gerity L., Anand, A. (Eds.) *The
Legacy of Edith Kramer*, Routledge London and New York, pp. 38–45.

Chapter 10

Art, death and mourning

The artist and art-psychotherapist perspective

Esther Dreifuss-Kattan

Artists: Howard Bass, Zizi Raymond and Esther Dreifuss-Kattan

This chapter will focus on using art and therapy with cancer patients in the later and terminal stage of cancer. When cancer patients are confronted with their terminal illness and there are no longer any treatments available, multiple mourning processes are activated, forcing both the patient and her therapist to make tremendous inner changes. Art making helps both the patient and her art-psychotherapist reflect on death and separation.

In the course of art therapy-psychotherapy of critically ill or dying cancer patients, an externalization of ego functions becomes necessary, as external relationships keep changing and the patient becomes weaker and is much more self-focused. Consequently, there is no resolution of the mutual relationships between patient and art therapist and great fears can be activated in both. The death of a patient still strongly enmeshed in a close relationship with the art-psychotherapist can cause a partial "death" in the therapist that she has to mourn as well.

Two short case vignettes of adult cancer patients—illustrated with dialogues and with their pictures—demonstrate the particular fears and concerns, both internal and external, that confronted them. Art is used both by the patient and art therapist to work through these intensely painful and often ambivalent losses that are followed by mourning for the deceased patient.

The Latin and Greek words for cancer present a paradox: While the Latin word for cancer is carcinoma, meaning tumor, the Greek word for cancer is neoplasm, translated as "forming of the new." The threat of destruction that this "new" cancerous tissue represents invariably evokes dread, but in many patients it also arouses new, formerly dormant creative energies, as the patients tap both physical and psychological resources to fight the illness. (Dreifuss-Kattan, 1990). As a patient struggles to restore their health and psychological balance after the trauma of a cancer diagnosis, a unique dialectic can emerge between illness and health and between despair and new hope. To this point, the Swiss author Walter Diggelman, who suffered from a brain tumor, wrote: "If my slow dying, which cannot be doubted any longer, is preordained, then I have only one last wish, that I can make out of it a beautiful, great exciting story" (Diggelman, 1979). Similarly, the British singer and composer David Bowie wrote the songs on his last album *Blackstar* (2016), and produced the music video for his song "Lazarus," after he became aware he was dying of cancer. The starkness and power of Bowie's style in his final work illustrates a new relationship to his art in light of his diagnosis. That is, though Bowie expressed himself creatively during his entire life, he felt a newly urgent need to work through his imminent death from cancer, treating his compositions as a memorial for his family and for his public. The work of mourning through creativity leads to a new perspective on reality, which manifests as a wish to continue living in order to create something in the present and for the future.

A diagnosis of cancer evokes anxieties, fears and grief and causes physical suffering, dependency and vulnerability. Cancer also allows the patient to focus on present experiences, as well as transforming her or his important interpersonal relationships, making reparation of inner and outer objects possible. From recent studies by Rodin et al. (2007), and from my own clinical experience, it is clear that hope and a will to live are preserved till the end of life in most cancer patients despite advanced, metastatic or terminal illness. Patients state that they want to continue living, in spite of the prospect of more pain and suffering. Nor do they want to anesthetize themselves by hastening a death their diagnosis makes inevitable (Breitbart et al., 2000). The awareness of death is experienced simultaneously with a wish to survive. Rodin and Zimmerman call this phenomenon a "middle knowledge" or "double awareness...in which states of awareness and denial may alternate, fluctuate and coexist ... evoking profound and contradictory emotions" (Rodin & Zimmermann, 2008, p. 186). I agree with Minerbo that it is very moving to witness the courage and dignity with which patients accept their own mortality, sometimes witnessing it face to face as well as through their art. (Minerbo 1998),

The confrontation with a potentially terminal illness like cancer forces the patient to make tremendous inner changes. On the narcissistic level, the patient must mourn the lost integrity of their own body or body function. This mourning is compounded by the aggressive assaults of invasive medical procedures, such as toxic chemotherapies with bad side effects, multiple surgeries, radiation treatments and other more targeted therapies. As a result, the patient often feels that their body and memory are degrading or even disintegrating. If we remember that the earliest development of the ego is closely connected with the image of an intact body ego, we can appreciate the threat to the feeling of self-worth, as well as the feelings of shame and anger that cancer can cause. The patient also begins to focus more intently on internal relationships and experiences from the past, as well as the reconstruction and interpretation of emotional and relational issues as they are accessed in the relationship with the art therapist in the present. Through this process, the patient in a terminal stage is able to withdraw the remaining good feelings and energy from his or her ailing body, thus allowing for a mourning process to unfold that can awaken amazing creative potential.

As patients find a new form of expression through art making, they elicit pleasurable and satisfying feelings in themselves despite the life-altering advent of cancer, and repair the narcissistic damage brought about by illness and treatments. The art they create can become a transformational object, a symbol that mediates between separation and togetherness and between dying and immortality. Artistic expression helps the cancer patient find new creative forms, as well as an encounter with an aesthetic moment, a satisfying and self-affirming experience, not unlike when one is looking at a very satisfying painting or sculpture in a museum. At the same time, cancer patients derive psychological insight from their art and put it to use working through life issues that were intractable before. From the perspective of the psychoanalyst/art therapist, the patient's artistic expression shows the psychological impact of therapy and disease, thus activating the analyst/therapist's counter-transference feelings toward the patient. I will illuminate these ideas with two case vignettes and some theoretical remarks.

Case vignette

I will first introduce you to Howard, a 69-year-old married man with one son and two grandchildren. A few years before I met Howard, his son was diagnosed with multiple myeloma and nearly died as a result of being treated with the wrong dose of chemotherapy. Howard's son spent three months in the intensive care unit with two collapsed lungs, nursed by his father and his stepmother, Howard's second wife, Michelle. His son recovered after two bouts of cancer and is now healthy.

Having gone through the trauma of his son's cancer and the diagnosis of his own cancer soon afterward, Howard projected to the group members and to me an adaptive denial, using excessive humor and sexual references to defend against his strong feelings of impotence. Howard's multiple myeloma was treated with chemotherapy and radiation that provided temporary relief, but a relapse eventually made stem cell transplantation necessary.

For three years, Howard was a member of two separate art/psychotherapy groups I facilitated for cancer patients of all ages and stages of illness at two different cancer centers. I therefore saw him often twice weekly for three years, with each group session lasting two hours. Because of our close bond, he developed a strong and positive transference relationship to me. Using Howard's art as an example, I would like to give a short illustration of some of the psychological issues that arise when a patient is faced with serious illness and its treatment and eventually, as in Howard's case, with death.

The powerful imagery of his work expresses the destructive process of cancer along with the restorative and reparative processes that are part

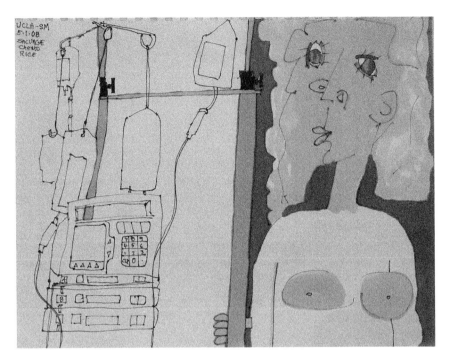

Figure 10.1 Howard Bass, "Salvage Chemo Ride," 2008.

of all artistic expressions. It exemplifies how the cancer patient reaches a longed-for transitional space between mother and infant, a space characterized by emotional support, creativity and play and a sense of expanding, infinite time (Figure 10.1).

The title describes the University of California Los Angeles Santa Monica hospital in which Howard was being treated. On the one side we see the monitor with its chemotherapy infusion bags, drawn in black and white. On the other, a pretty, blonde, sexy nurse with very blue eyes and cute, perky pink breasts is depicted. The title suggests that when Howard focuses on the nurse's breasts, the scary, dehumanizing chemotherapy ride is not so bad. The nurse looks very similar to his wife Michelle, upon whom he can depend, as she is a loving support to him. Distracted and buoyed by his sexual fantasies, Howard manages to soldier on through his fears of chemotherapy (Figure 10.2).

This colorful scene depicts three naked adults. In the middle we see a woman who seems like Howard's wife looking straight at us. On one side, we see our patient Howard, in a kind of self-portrait, wearing a white undershirt with his penis uncovered. On the other side we find a thin, vulnerable, completely naked bald man who looks down. The red fire hydrant

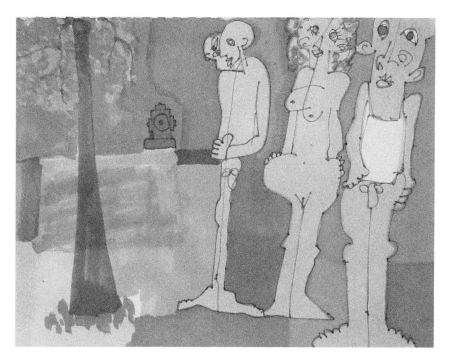

Figure 10.2 Howard Bass, "Untitled," 2008.

looms in the background. We can interpret the scene as Howard's ambivalent awareness of his situation: he feels healthy and strong in one image,
but vulnerable and sickly in the other. The two realities are surfacing unconsciously, but as they begin to appear on paper, Howard is confronted
by the paradox of his self-image. The red fire hydrant speaks to his wish
to receive help in order to extinguish the "cancer fire" that seems to be
spreading (Figure 10.3).

Howard portrays himself in the middle of a group of vulnerable, sick,
naked adults. His use of a thin pen makes this feeling of helplessness very
prominent. These people or patients all seem very worried. He identifies
with all his fellow cancer patients, like the ones in the "Cancer and Creativity" group he attends, for instance, who can understand and empathize
with his challenges. The support of his peers allows him to observe himself
and others, and to acknowledge his sadness, his fear of death and his great
physical and emotional defenselessness (Figure 10.4).

This colorful picture compellingly renders Howard's closeness to his
wife and supporters and the hope he felt at the time he drew it. Howard
(with bald head due to chemotherapy) and his wife-mother-therapist are
contained in one basket that moves up into the sky. The basket is filled

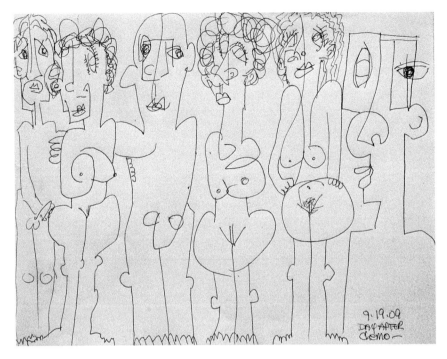

Figure 10.3 Howard Bass, "Day After Chemo," 2009.

with hope and wishes for good health. It also contains the blessings for his family, art therapy (the relationship with his art therapist and the pleasure of art making) and medication. Howard is not alone, his basket is full, and while his companion seems worried, she is also definitively present (Figure 10.5).

Both titles explain Howard's situation very well. While Howard portrays himself in one corner with a woman, possibly representing his wife, as well as his therapist in the transference, he also holds open the coffin lid that he suggests is not for him, but for his ex-wife. His ex-wife is the mother of his son, and Howard still projects onto her his dissatisfying relationship with her, as well as an estranged relationship with his long-dead mother. The street sign directs us to the cemetery and a desperate Howard is standing on the brown surface of shit/dirt, while there still seems to be a potential escape to the greener grass on the other side or out of the window toward the blue sky. The patient would like to shut the coffin on his bad internal objects— his aggressive father and unloving mother, who still fill him with rage. He realizes that time is running out, which he illustrates by drawing his legs already half inside the brown dirt, thus implying that he is being slowly buried. The patient becomes aware that the rage he projects toward his dead

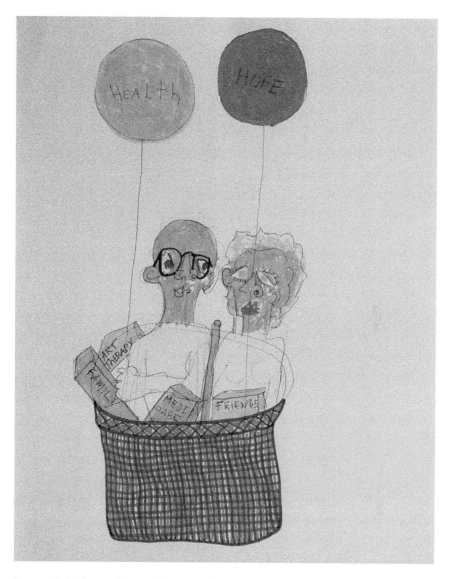

Figure 10.4 Howard Bass, "Basket of Blessings," 2009.

parents belongs partly to the destructive cancer that leaves him furious and impotent. He is sad in spite of his very good and caring oncologist and his devoted wife and art therapist, who all love him very much and admire his artistic talents and his humor. All their support, however, cannot stop the progression of his cancer (Figures 10.6 and 10.7).

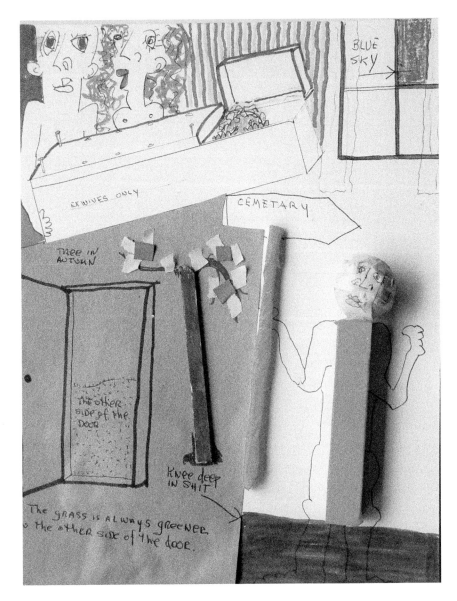

Figure 10.5 Howard Bass, "Knee Deep in Shit," 2009.

Prior to Howard's painting this image, I prompted the group members to make a self-portrait first and then another portrait of somebody who came to mind. After Howard painted his self-portrait, he explained that the second portrait was of me, his art therapist. I came to his mind, he explained, because he needed to talk to me. I did not know what he had

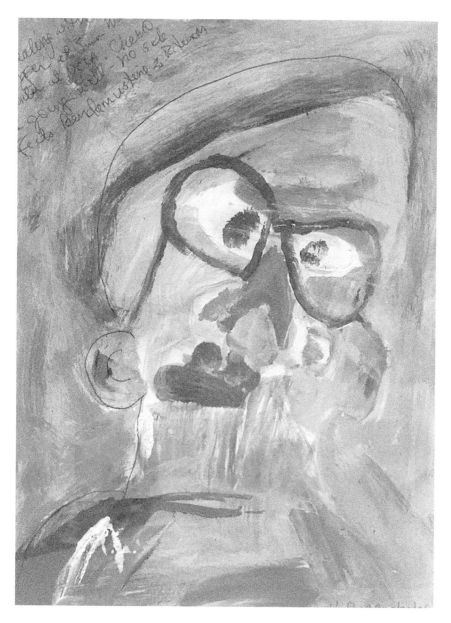

Figure 10.6 Howard Bass, "Two Portraits: A Dialog," 2009.

planned to communicate to me, as after this "Cancer and Creativity" group ended, Howard suddenly had to be admitted to the Intensive Care Unit in the University Hospital. He was hooked up to many life-saving machines when I came to visit as he had requested, and he was too weak to talk, so he

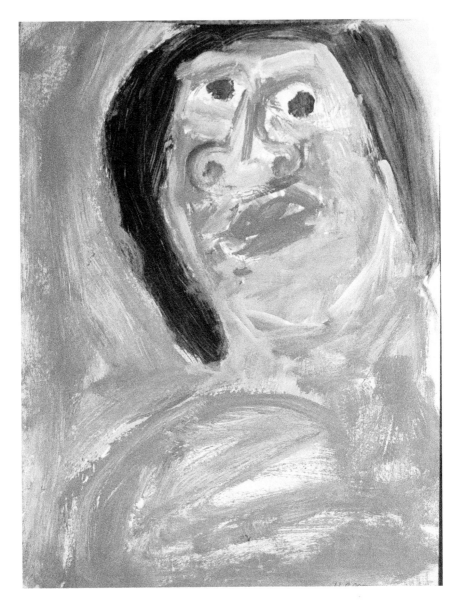

Figure 10.7 Howard Bass, "Two Portraits: A Dialog," 2009.

carefully and slowly wrote out a dialog with me on his laptop. He wrote that he did not want to die; he wanted to live longer because he was not done living yet. I suddenly realized why he had wanted to talk to me after the group. He wrote that he felt calm, but very sad, then made eye contact with me and asked what I was thinking. I replied that he must feel that death was close, but that he had not yet given up hope and neither had I. I pointed out to him that he had touched many people in his life and during his cancer journey; he had forged strong and loving ties with his oncologist/father, his son, his wife, fellow patients in the group and with me. We admired his courage and his wit, an admiration which moved his wife to express so much love and care for him. He then asked me if he should go home to die, as his wife wished, but which his doctors were trying to prevent. As I realized he had become reconciled to his fate, I recalled to him that he always hated being in the hospital for too long and that if he felt more comfortable at home in his apartment overlooking the Pacific Ocean, I was certain that this would be a good option for him. When his wife returned after our session, they decided together to go home the next day. On his way out of his hospital bed the following morning, Howard passed away in the presence of his beloved wife.

After each group session and then after the ICU visit, I was deeply moved and emotionally overwhelmed. I would take a few minutes outside his room to gather myself emotionally, as I mourned Howard while he still was alive and at the same time still mourned my mother, who had died less than a year earlier. Howard's pictures and transitional objects provided him and me as well with an acceptable defense to navigate our therapeutic encounter. Once he was hospitalized, however, no defense mechanism was strong enough for Howard or for me. It was a great privilege to share Howard and Michelle's journey to the end of his life.

Art-psychotherapy work with terminal cancer patients

In the course of art-psychotherapy with seriously ill and dying cancer patients, an externalization of ego function slowly becomes necessary as personal relationships change and eventually become reduced. The closer the patient is to death, the more he or she focuses on himself or herself, redirecting psychic and somatic energies toward survival. Consequently, a traditional resolution of transference cannot occur in many cases, provoking fear in both the patient and the therapist. When the patient dies while still strongly enmeshed in the relationship to the therapist, the mourning therapist experiences a partial death within herself.

An idealized transference to the empathic therapist can develop in a later stage of illness, as the patient wishes to regress to a very early condition of love, total security and absolute trust. Handling the ambivalence that is inherent in any idealization can be a challenge. Often, while in the first phase of regression because of illness, patients imagine the art therapist as an idealized parental imago or an equally idealized punishing and neglecting one. The psychotherapist, due to her perceived good health and vitality, can quickly find herself in the role of the envied parent, sibling or friend and thus rejected by the cancer patient out of consequent negative effects of anger, disillusionment and envy. Rejecting the therapist often represents the only way for the very sick person faced with cancer to appease his or her judging super ego. Stopping treatment at a time when the patient needs the most support, therefore, becomes his or her attempt to ward off guilty feelings, a sense of shame and a fear of being rejected or abandoned later on. (Schaverien, 1999)

Spero (2004) movingly discusses a woman with breast cancer who during psychoanalytic psychotherapy spontaneously expressed religious metaphors, revealing new layers of memory. The psychoanalyst, listening and recognizing his counter-transference feelings even without verbalizing them, helped the patient to rediscover "a sacred healing breast," reconnecting her to the religious experiences from her early childhood and allowing her to reactivate a new sense of time that resulted in new meaning.

In a later phase of treatment, as the cancer relapses or progresses, the therapist is often forced to take over more of the ego functions, as well as to try to balance a new therapeutic framework. Norton (1963) started to read to her patient with cancer when she became blind. A need might arise to see the patients in their homes, or speak to them on the telephone, as they become too weak to come to the office or to the outpatient clinic. This new, more essentially maternal connection can help the patient to perceive the therapist as more internally present, even when he or she is absent. Because of the greater dependency of the cancer patient on the art therapist, the mutual relationship can become particularly emotionally intense. Eissler (1973) believes the strong bond is necessary, as it relieves suffering, despite pain caused by the progressively deteriorating somatic process. The intense, sometimes also erotic, transference mobilizes an archaic trust that reawakens the essential feelings of parental protection. In a fascinating case study, Schaverien (1999) discusses a patient with depression who was in analysis with her when he was diagnosed with inoperable lung cancer. Being faced with death, an even more intense, dependent and erotic transference developed that challenged boundary issues of the therapeutic encounter. During the course of psychotherapeutic treatment, her patient was able to move from more defensive adult sexual Oedipal feelings to more pre-Oedipal ones, enabling an individuation process—despite his terminal illness—from dependency to self-reliance. He was able to finally move out of his parents' home, enabling him to die as a middle-aged man under the care and support of his adult sister. His newfound independence allowed his father to share with his dying son his great sorrow of losing him too soon.

One feature of a primary partnership between a cancer patient and an art therapist or psychotherapist, as mentioned earlier and as seen in Howard's case, is that the relationship is always threatened by an impending loss and thus has to be preserved at all times. Hence it has ambivalent characteristics. Both patient and therapist feel the wish to withdraw, so as to anticipate separation, and the opposing wish to cling, in order to avoid separation. Again, both these tendencies are true for patient as well as therapist.

Case vignette

Sabine, a long-term breast cancer survivor and artist, participated in my Healing Arts Support groups for several years. Sabine was a talented artist and loved the group's structure with its social support and art making during a set time every week. The sicker she became, the more important this link to drawing and painting and the group members became.

Sabine was the middle child between a brother and a sister, and her late father was involved in a creative profession. She often talked to her aunt, who was interested in her art making and provided stability in her early life.

Sabine showed up in our group often immediately after some medical intervention or important treatments or upsetting doctor appointments. She seemed unfazed through these invasive treatments, animated with a force of life and unable to be barred from spending a couple hours from art making. She was goal-oriented, focused and always ready to work. While she listened carefully to my particular instructions each week, she also felt quite comfortable ignoring some of my weekly ideas, an autonomy I encouraged.

Sabine, like some other members of the group, used her iPhone as an aid to remember the themes I suggested and the practical art instructions in the beginning of each of the group sessions as her health problems expanded, from memory loss to impaired mobility. Losing her freedom of movement disappointed her and added to her burdens, emphasizing the progression of her cancer. In spite of her medical issues and limitations she remained a very active and independent person. She had grown accustomed to visiting friends, going to markets, galleries, museums and restaurants with friends or alone.

I liked Sabine and admired her strength and creativity, as well as her fortitude in the face of her reoccurring Lymphoma for several years. I did not want her now to miss out on the "Healing Arts" group, and thus decided with others that we would pick her up for the group meetings when my schedule allowed it.

As our therapeutic relationship within the group setting expanded to a friendship or caregiver, based on our mutual interest in art and my care for her, I realized that I needed to take over some of her ego function and become helpful beyond the art therapy group setting. As her cancer progressed, her close friends in the group and I became more worried about her living alone, not eating enough and her unsettling future, something we felt was barely addressed on a practical level by her doctors. While I realized that what I had begun to offer Sabine extended beyond a more traditional therapeutic relationship of an art therapist to a patient in a therapeutic group, I still kept a therapeutic framework intact. I attended instead to her needs and concerns more, holding her when we walked and encouraging her to eat. I recognized how necessary and pleasing it was for Sabine to still be actively involved in the creative world of the arts, outside of the "Cancer and Creativity" group and her active cancer world.

One afternoon over lunch, after Sabine shared with me that she had fallen recently while alone in her home, I gingerly started a discussion about her future, when she would need more consistent care and help. Sabine was taken aback initially and wondered if I was overreacting, but at the same time was grateful for my suggestions and became more quiet and thoughtful. We started to discuss plans for the future and I suggested that she needed to share her issues, with her brother and sister.

Sabine must have felt confused, as I had blurred the boundaries inherent to being her group art psychotherapist by also addressing some very practical issues: I was thus less equipped to deliver bad news and to pierce the strong adaptive defense that had served her so well for the past 10 years. Indeed, like her family I had begun to feel a personal responsibility to ensure she would not be alone when she will get weaker or more vulnerable to unnecessary physical suffering and psychological trauma. Sabine's family had respected her wish for total independence up to this point, but as she entered the more terminal stage her brother and sister began to take charge of her care with much love and kindness.

After our exchange about her future over lunch, Sabine initially reconciled with me and was happy to see me when I visited her in the hospital. As she grew weaker and sicker and closer to death, however, she withdrew from me, even when I came to wait outside her hospital room until she woke up. I realized that toward the end of life most dying patients reduce their emotional involvement to a few good friends and close family members, as they need to focus on themselves to conserve the few energies they still command. But, unconsciously, my active, therapeutic intervention that time over lunch might have made the patient feel that I had pushed her too much toward facing her own death, trampling over and exposing the denial that served her well up to this point. Sabine perhaps, could not fully forgive me for that.

The "Healing Arts" group had offered this artist with cancer a new encounter with art and art making, an occupation she was fully and very successfully engaged in during her short healthy adult life. Her participation in the group upheld and strengthened her identity as an artist, and as a productive person in spite of terminal cancer.

Zizi's circles

You met the artist Zizi Raymond in chapter 2 and in chapter 6. We curated several art exhibitions over the five years when she was in the groups. Zizi was often featured alone or as part of a group exhibition. She would select works, and even hang the art, depending on her physical strength at that time.

During the last two years of her life Zizi repeatedly painted, drew or made collages of circles. The circle pieces are in all different sizes and colors; some are painted with acrylic paint, but for most Zizi used Swiss-made Caran'Dache Neocolor water-soluble crayons. In the collages, she would cut circles out of random magazines or fabric. The pieces have different color combinations, and the shapes of the circles vary: sometimes perfectly round, sometimes more oval or ringlike. The variations in size and composition, I believe, depended on Zizi's mood and health status. When we talked about the circle pictures, Zizi named them as "blood cells," "cancer cells," "feces," "a color palette" or "just round shapes" depending on the stage of her symptoms and health status and her mood or level of suffering. Indeed, Zizi seemed totally engrossed when painting or crafting her circles and barely participated in the less significant communicative acts going on in the room around her, like our group discussion. Hence, we could read psychological insights disclosed by that week's color choices and particular forms (Figure 10.8).

Looking at Zizi's many circle paintings, we might see the circle as an organic or biological metaphor of an internal universe or connect it to Zizi's suffering from breast cancer, whose symbol is two circles. These curving, encompassing shapes might have been her way to gather in solidarity all of her other cancer-patient friends in the "Cancer and Creativity" group and other groups, enfolding members into whole family constellations. Circles also denote backward and forward movement as they curve back on themselves, making them images with a particular unconscious essence: outlining and coloring them seemed for this artist a kind of meditation. (Derrida, 1987) Using circles as a theme might have been Zizi's way of retracing her steps, marking the edges, securing an aesthetic, somatic, regulative and rhythmic experience in the context of living with the acute anxieties provoked by metastatic breast cancer and approaching death. It might have been her way of interweaving different threads of her life, provoked by a desire for restitution and integration, as well as a playful game of inside and outside, background and foreground, stranger and friend. The duality of inside and outside is also recognized in the workings of the body with its challenged organs and physiology, and with the internally perceived vulnerable and helpless self with and fear of death.

Traditional art making and a transitional art career were impossible for this cancer patient who—in addition to multiple metastases and recurrences

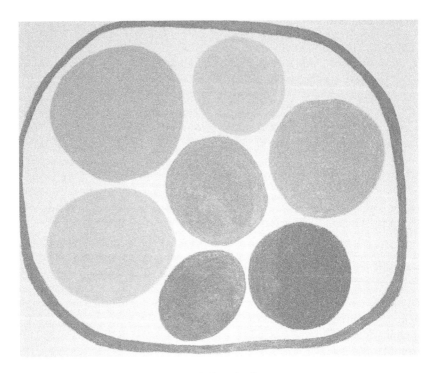

Figure 10.8 Zizi Raymond: "Circles," Acrylic Paint.

of her breast cancer for so many years—was treated with unconventional and unusually intrusive surgeries. A Whipple procedure was done to remove tumors from her pancreas, and she endured multiple laser brain surgeries, radiation treatments, chemotherapy sessions and clinical trials of new drugs. The "Cancer and Creativity" group provided the formal and material means for this talented artist to reinvent herself as an artist once again, in the company of other artists who shared different but similar cancer journeys (Figures 10.9 and 10.10).

Countertransference in the art therapist

The following short case vignette illustrates the countertransference issues in the psychotherapist and the great ambivalence these issues can engender. The dying patient can mobilize in the psychotherapist her own childish death wishes and the psychotherapist can be reminded of her own mortality. We know well that when one of our patients dies, we also have to mourn the loss and have to deal with our own survivor's guilt. This guilt together with the dying patient's envy or even hatred toward the surviving therapist can be a great burden. One of the main defenses the psychooncologist unconsciously

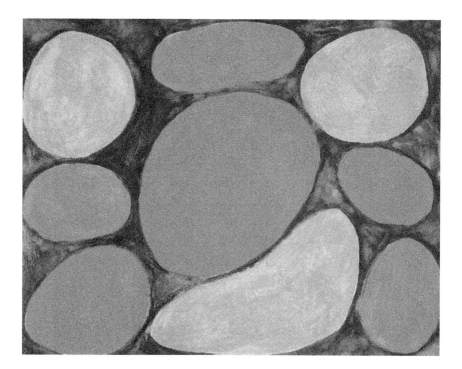

Figure 10.9 Zizi Raymond: "Circles," Acrylic Paint.

employs is a heightened sense of identification with the dying patient, which is eased by mobilizing various distancing mechanisms. These defenses, stimulated by the countertransference, can be expressed in various ways, such as missing sessions or trying to calm the patient with superficial comments, becoming overprotective or overintellectualizing the therapeutic dialog or encounter. Such unconscious defenses aim at overcoming the great ambivalence the therapist feels toward merging with the seriously or terminally ill patient. These feelings of ambivalence cannot really be fully worked through, and they are inherent in working with seriously ill and dying cancer patients. However, if the art therapist becomes consciously aware of them, she can prevent their being acted out destructively with the patient. (Dreifuss-Kattan, 1990)

Case vignette

I worked for nearly three years in psychoanalytic psychotherapy with Emma, a single, 42-year-old woman who was an editor in a well-known publishing company. Emma had been suffering from breast cancer for five years and had undergone numerous operations and difficult chemotherapy and radiation treatments. We had established an excellent rapport, with the frequency

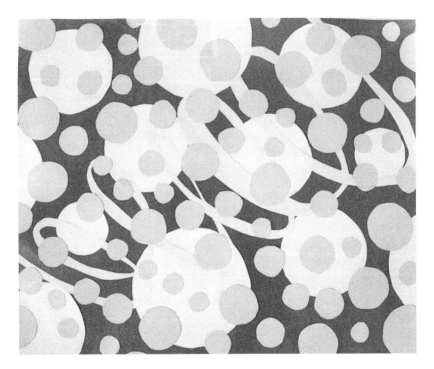

Figure 10.10 Zizi Raymond: "Circles," Acrylic Paint.

and nature of our sessions altering with the state of her illness. With the help of psychotherapy, the patient found different means of expressing herself when her longstanding wish to write reasserted itself toward the end of her life. She was thankful toward me for having helped her to attain this goal. Yet she also envied my good health, my professional position and my independence and autonomy. I could all too easily identify with her. We were close in age, both single at that time and had the same artistic and cultural interests. The more ill the patient became, the closer, and, at the same time, the more ambivalent our relationship grew. On one hand, I represented to Emma the healthy and creative parts of her own personality. On the other hand, I was a mirror through which she saw the limitations of her own life and her forthcoming death. Even though she attained some success with her literary publications, she increasingly realized that her creativity could not halt the malignant process of her cancer, as she unconsciously fantasized.

Supplementing intensive psychoanalytic supervision, I had a need to make paintings of Emma in my free time at home, in an attempt to work through and mourn this intense relationship. I used acrylic paint and stretched canvas for my pictures. When I started to paint, the patient was

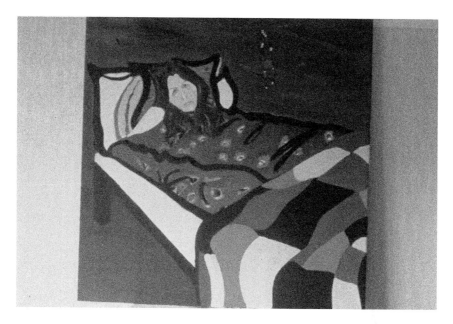

Figure 10.11 Esther Dreifuss-Kattan: "In Bed," Acrylic on Canvas, 1989. These last paintings were previously published in Cancer Stories: Creativity and Self-Repair (The Analytic Press, Hillsdale NY, 1990).

already in the terminal phase of her illness and I was visiting her in her home. (Dreifuss-Kattan, 1990) (Figure 10.11).

I painted the patient realistically, lying in her bed. Her imploring look might be saying, "Come, Esther, do something for me." Both her position and her expression reflected her actual conduct. She looks in my painting not unlike me; unconsciously I must have expressed my identification with Emma. Over her bed hung a small red wooden toy, which represented for me her cancer, as it looked like a small crab. Whenever I arrived for our twice-weekly session, Emma was happy to see me, eager to share her writing and associations with me, but at the same time quick to communicate her frustration that whatever I had to give her was not good enough. Unconsciously she might have wanted more: my healthy body, maybe, and what she fantasized about as my unlimited future (Figure 10.12).

In this painting I emphasized the more seductive, provocative quality of Emma. She seems to fight flirtatiously with Death, who is trying to push her down. As I looked at this picture, I came to realize for the first time that I felt strongly that Emma was trying to draw me in, to seduce me with an invitation to death, as though she were saying: "See, it's not all that bad, just join me." This emerging erotic transference and wish for fusion made me very uncomfortable (Figure 10.13).

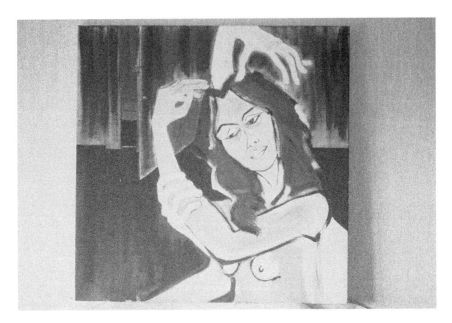

Figure 10.12 Esther Dreifuss-Kattan: "Flirting With Death," Acrylic Paint on Canvas, 1989. These last paintings were previously published in Cancer Stories: Creativity and Self-Repair (The Analytic Press, Hillsdale NY, 1990).

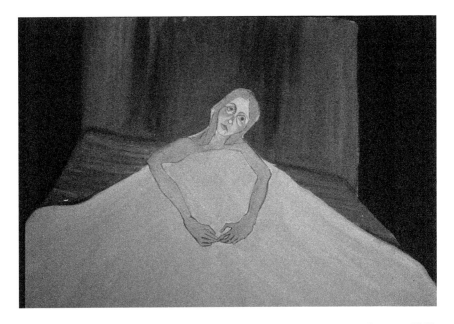

Figure 10.13 Esther Dreifuss-Kattan: "Distance," Acrylic Paint on Canvas, 1989. These last paintings were previously published in Cancer Stories: Creativity and Self-Repair (The Analytic Press, Hillsdale NY, 1990).

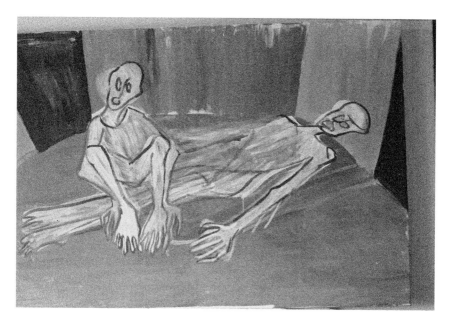

Figure 10.14 Esther Dreifuss-Kattan: "Identification," Acrylic Paint on Canvas, 1989. These last paintings were previously published in Cancer Stories: Creativity and Self-Repair (The Analytic Press, Hillsdale NY, 1990).

My wish for distancing manifests itself in my portrayal of Emma's bed, as is clear from the perspective I drew. Emma now lies alone in her bed and seems to be hiding something under her blanket. In our sessions, Emma was beginning to talk more and more about her wish to commit suicide and asked me to facilitate this process. I interpreted her suicidal wishes as a desire to take her fate into her own hands, to regain control over her life, death and destiny and to become independent of her caregivers. At the same time, I told her I could not be of any assistance in this act, as the law did not allow it at that time in the place she lived. Our visits became more and more difficult, and I resisted how the patient wanted to draw me into her suicidal intentions. The pressure that I felt must have inspired my fourth and last painting (Figure 10.14).

In a virtual rage, I painted for eight hours, putting color over color in an all-day battle on a big two-meter canvas. I was shocked by the result. There I am, sitting on the patient's stiff, dead body—a corpse myself, fully identi-fied with her. I realized how eager I was on an unconscious level to have this patient pass away, to be done with her coaxing and cajoling, with her intense suffering and her longing to die that had made me feel so very guilty. I felt so guilty that I had turned her into a corpse before her time and I transformed myself into a corpse as well. It was as though I felt that only by dying myself could I attain a guilt-free peace of mind after our very close and meaningful but long and painful journey together. (Dreifuss-Kattan, 1990)

I had to act out my own death wishes on a creative level, recognizing my own countertransference as I did, before I could accompany Emma to the end of her life without acting out my aggression within our therapeutic encounter or by assisting her suicidal intention. I recognized the power of the psychotherapist's ambivalence only in my own paintings. They enabled me to gain control over my ambivalent feelings without mobilizing unconscious defenses, allowing me to treat Emma on her deathbed with empathy and an open mind. (Dreifuss-Kattan, 1990)

Art making, be it with color and paint, with musical composition or poetry and writing, allows for the externalization and transformation of strong feelings of loss. Art is a powerful tool for the caregivers as well, generative of strong insights, illuminative of one's own unconscious feelings toward our dying patients, especially when combined with professional mourning rituals. Learning to read and interpret one's own creative expression can facilitate our own mourning process and leaves behind a memorial that reminds us of a life that has been lost.

References

Breitbart, W., et al. (2000). Depression, hopelessness, and the desire for hastened death in terminally ill patients with cancer. *Journal of the American Medical Association, 284,* 2907–2911.

Derrida, J. (1987). *The Truth in Painting*, Trans. Bennington G. and McLeod I. Chicago IL: University of Chicago Press.

Diggelman, W. (1979). *Schatten, Tagebuch einer Krankheit [Shadows, Diary of an Illness].* Zuerich: Benzinger.

Dreifuss-Kattan, E. (1990). *Cancer Stories: Creativity and Self Repair.* Hillsdale, NJ: The Analytic Press.

Eissler, K. (1973). *The Psychiatrist and the Dying Patient.* New York: International University Press.

Minerbo, V. (1998). The patient without a couch: An analysis of a patient with terminal cancer. *International Journal of Psycho-Analysis, 79* (1), 83–93.

Norton, J. (1963). *Treatment of a Dying Patient. The Psychoanalytic Study of the Child.* New York: International University Press. 25, 360–400

Rodin, G., et al. (2007) Treatment of depression in Cancer patients. *Current Oncology, 14* (5).

Rodin, G., & Zimmermann, C. (2008). Psychoanalytic reflection on mortality: Reconsideration. *Journal of American Academy of Psychoanalysis and Dynamic Psychotherapy, 36* (1), 181–196.

Schaverien, J. (1999). The death of an analysand: Transference, countertransference and desire. *Journal of Analytical Psychology, 44* (1), 3–28.

Spero, M. H. (2004). Hearing the faith in time: Countertransference and religious metaphor in an oncology patient's psychotherapy. *Psychoanalytic Quarterly, 73* (4), 971–1021.

Chapter 11

Art and cancer in the public space

Suzanne Isken

From April to June 2013, Esther Dreifuss-Kattan curated an exhibition of work by five artists, most of whom were participating in her "Cancer and Creativity" group. The exhibition was entitled "From the Canvas to the Couch: Art and Cancer" and was staged at the New Center for Psychoanalysis in Los Angeles. It featured an opening reception and lecture with an accompanying modest catalog. The exhibition was open to the public and attracted family and friends of the artists as well as students and institute members attending meetings and events at the center. This exhibit serves as the basis for many of the observations shared here about viewing and exhibiting art about cancer. As the cocurator of the exhibition, I consulted with the artists to arrange their work into a cohesive story that highlighted each individual. As always in a group show featuring diverse media, including sculpture, installation, photography and works on paper, the challenge is to make the works fit together visually. Solving this problem for a group show of artists with cancer is not so different from solving it for artists without cancer: the legislation of gallery real estate is always a minefield that must be sensitively negotiated. Artists care about the gallery lighting, how the wall labels reflect their identity and whether or not their work is visible in, and through, the context of the group.

An artist's self-image is always vulnerable when their work is in front of the public, but artists are generally proud and optimistic about their chance to communicate with a wider audience. Artists usually express that they expect their work to stand on its own, communicating something that is more fundamental than any initial inspiration in their own biographies. In fact, even the artists' conception of what inspired their work, or where it came from, can change over time, as expressed by artist Corrine Lightweaver in the "From the Canvas to the Couch: Art and Cancer" catalog. Lightweaver remarked that she was surprised by the changes in her artist statements she wrote after she had acquired some temporal distance from the work. Her writing became more detached over time, changing first-person statements to third-person references in the accompanying text.

To understand the importance of exhibiting the artwork of people with cancer or cancer survivors, I would propose to answer first the question of why artists exhibit work about their cancer experiences, before moving on to how the public engages with art exhibitions and to the conclusions we can draw from this interplay of artist and audience. I will propose an interpretive approach to take when viewing art by cancer patients and offer suggestions for creating opportunities for public dialogue about cancer during the course of an exhibition.

The contemporary idea of art as a healing process was firmly established by artist Joseph Bueys after World War II. Born in 1921, Bueys served as a Hitler Youth before crashing his airplane in Crimea in 1943 while serving in the Luftwaffe (Nazi Air Force), an experience that would prove transformative for him. The story goes that Bueys was rescued by nomadic Tartars who lived in the region, who picked up his wounded body from the snow and covered him with a layer of fat, then wrapped him in felt, carried him on a sledge and nursed him back to health using traditional and shamanistic rituals of healing. Bueys' convalescence with the Tartars was revelatory for him, leading him to believe in the potential for universal peace between differing ethnic groups and leading to a dramatic career shift toward art. Specifically, Bueys began to conceive of art as a healing process and a metaphor for transforming Western education, politics and economic systems.

After his return to Germany, Bueys joined the Dusseldorf Academy of Art to study sculpture, but also joined the Fluxus movement, a group of artists who rejected the idea of art as the expression of an individual ego, and sought to transgress all boundaries between art and life in their work. Fluxus existed as a community of friends who experimented together to create new forms of art and expression. Bueys took from Fluxus teachings that every human being is an artist, since everyone possesses creative faculties that must be identified and developed. He associated creativity with resurrection and expanded art into a way of living that cultivates life, soul and spirit, a capacious mission Bueys intended for the "evolutionary-revolutionary power" of art. Bueys' practice included making sculptural objects, installations and creating public performances called "Actions," such as "I Like America, America Likes Me" (1974), in which Bueys lived in a cage with a wild coyote for three days. The piece imagines the coyote as a scapegoat, a detested animal burdened with projections of American feelings of inferiority and with racist antipathy toward Native Americans. By confronting this animal in a type of forced "dialogue," Bueys becomes a spiritual healer, whose shamanic affinity with animals allows him to enact a symbolic reconciliation between modern American society, the natural world and Native American culture, all on American soil where the piece was staged. His performances offered dramatic lessons aimed to demonstrate to everyone the healing potential of art. He felt these Actions were a kind of therapy.

In his installations and sculptures, Bueys incorporated discarded bloody bandages, broken pill bottles, rusty syringes, old medical textbooks, animal bones, radiography films and other medical artifacts. The metaphor of the wound encompasses his emotional state, spiritual state and a politically divided world; works are entitled *Woman with Head Bandage, Bleeding Stag*, and *Show Your Wound*. The wound also counteracts the fascist notion of beautifying everything, the famous fascist "aestheticization of politics" as described by Walter Benjamin meshing with the enduringly debated notion in aesthetics proper that art must be beautiful. Many contemporary artists have long shunned beauty as a falsehood that hides the painful reality of the real world. Beauty is no longer associated purely with goodness or value and artists maintain their insistence that illustrating raw emotion, rifts, wounds and nightmares can undermine the sense that only beauty represents the importance of being human._By concentrating on art as a healing practice, as opposed to beautification, Bueys expanded the notion of what could be considered art and who could be considered an artist. Leaving a solitary studio practice behind, Bueys turned to lectures, performances and public sculpture as the methods of healing; in a way that may be ambiguous—we may be unsure who is being healed, artist or audience—he posits that art as therapy depends on full-time engagement with other human beings.

Art created explicitly as a healing process has been an important branch of contemporary art practice since the 1940s, and for many artists diagnosed with cancer, their art production has been both personal and political. One of the most well-known feminist artists of her time was Hannah Wilke, an eventual cancer patient, whose work from the 1970s to 1980s exposes and dwells on the female body. Wilke, herself stunningly beautiful, radically unclothed herself and flaunted her body to make erotic art with vaginal imagery in feminist performances, mocking the idea of female beauty as an artistic and intellectual muse. She often made visual references to the art historical depictions of Venus/Aphrodite by mimicking the artificial poses, but making them more sexually explicit than their well-known European painting counterparts. Some art historians like Lippard criticized Wilke for confusing her role as a glamorous object of desire with her role a feminist. Wilke's diagnosis and treatment, however, and subsequent work recast this earlier period, as she maintained the photographic focus on her body to catalogue its ravaging and physical deterioration. The contrast with her idealized perfection as a socially defined female beauty is sharp.

Wilke's *Intra-Venus 1990–1993* documents her last three years of life while she was treated for lymphoma. She maintains her image as a Venus alter ego, but surgical bandages, hair loss and dwindling muscle tone begin to transform her appearance. In a set of video tapes, 14 years in the making and completed after her death according to her instructions, *Intra-Venus 1990–1993* shows the artist as she travels through stages of cheer, bodily deterioration and ends in a comatose state. Wilke constructs her legacy by focusing on the creation of her final work until her last moments of breath.

While making these final works was important to Wilke in the context of coping with cancer and maintaining her identity as an artist during her cancer years, the exhibition of this work was essential to her. She exhibited the work, just as she exhibited a similar documentation of her mother's battle with cancer (*So Help Me Hannah: Portrait of the Artist with her Mother Selma Butter 1978–1981*), in order to confront clinical procedures that hide patients as if dying was a personal shame. Wilke, on the contrary, wanted to construct an apparent, perceptible testimony via the photographs and videos, which would in turn endure as a legacy. Wilke asks the viewer to "witness what cancer has been like for me." Through her photography she admonishes us not to look away, as she cannot look away.

More recently, in June 2016, 31-year-old, New York artist Kaylin Andres articulately explained the importance of exhibiting her art work about cancer this way:

> I am an artist and writer diagnosed with a rare form of bone cancer called Ewing's Sarcoma. This is an attempt to document my process and provide inspiration for other twenty-somethings who refuse to go the way of headscarves and hospital gowns. I mean, really? Cancer is fucking hilarious.

Andres' exhibition at the Jenn Singer Gallery in New York in 2016 followed eight years of radiation, chemotherapy and surgery that coincided with her art production and advocacy for young adults with cancer. Her background in fashion design informed her visual art work, which combined photography with textiles embroidered with hair lost from the side effects of chemotherapy and handmade reliquaries inspired by her own spiritual journey of healing and survival. Andres' exhibition was entitled "Viaticum," the name for the receiving of the Eucharist before death: the last rites. The exhibition of her work, following its creation, served as a healing process that sustained her spirit. Andres firmly believed that to make art is to take from one's inner world and make it material—to give it life in the physical realm.

Another motivation for creating and exhibiting work was articulated by artist Lavialle Campbell whose exhibition at Coagula Curatorial in Los Angeles (May 27–July 2, 2017) was entitled *In the Shadows*. In an interview with curator Matt Gleason, Campbell explains that the hand-stitched quilts she made about her experience with breast cancer stemmed from her need "to purge from my system things about my health over the years." For Campbell, making and exhibiting this body of work created a sense of closure, a split between "now" and "then." This closure contrasted with work created in clay at an earlier stage of her journey as a cancer survivor.

Art writer Derrick (2017) further describes Campbell's quilts: "working with shades of indigo, purple, gray, and black, with impacts of acid yellow green, Campbell stitches together her experiences: gender, race, survivor of multiple life-threatening illnesses, artist." Derrick reminds us that when an artist with cancer makes work about cancer, the work reflects so much more about the person than their illness alone. Once exhibited, art can provoke the viewer to examine their own reactions to gender, race, illness and mortality; they too might emerge transformed. The viewer can begin to understand the gravity of cancer in its place, as only one part of a life experience transformed in unpredictable ways.

To that point, as mentioned earlier, art about cancer need not pass up being political. Two remarkable artists whose fight with cancer was associated with their initial diagnosis of HIV/AIDs were David Wojnarowicz and Felix Gonzales Torres. Wojnarowicz died of AIDS in 1992 at 37. In the late 1980s he described his life: "I'm in the throes of facing my own mortality and in attempting to communicate what I'm expressing or learning in order to try and help others" (Interview 2012 with Cynthia Carr, p.1). Wojnarowicz was insistent that he be recognized as a gay male, as an AIDS patient and as a human being. His art bridges contradictory desires for his personal experience to be recognized as such and for it to catalyze a sense of community between others grappling with illness. For Wojnarowicz, in other words, the personal was political, and the public's unwillingness to see the ravages of AIDS made it impossible to exert the political pressure needed to find a cure. Creating art about AIDS became a way to advocate for better and more humane research and the allocation of resources toward finding a cure.

Felix Gonzales Torres exhibited his work for similar reasons, stating "my work is my personal history…I can't separate my art from my life" (1993 interview with Rollins.). A work by Torres called *Untitled (Perfect Lovers) 1987–90*, the dates his lover was sick and dying, involves two synchronized clocks. The artist stated that the piece was important to him as it faced the issues of time and mortality, but added: "I want the public to feel…I want the public to be informed, moved to action." Gonzales Torres then elaborates on why exhibition is so important to his art about his personal experience. "Perhaps between public and private," he offers,

> between personal and social, between the fear of loss and the joy of loving, of growing, of changing, of always becoming more, of losing oneself slowly and then being replenished all over again from scratch. I need the viewer, I need public interaction. Without a public these works are nothing, nothing. I need the public to complete my work. I ask the public to help me, to take responsibility, to become part of my work, to join in. I tend to think of myself as a theater director who is trying to convey some ideas by reinterpreting the notion of the division of roles: author, public, and director
>
> (Interview with Rollins, 1993)

The artists featured in the "From the Canvas to the Couch" exhibition, like the artists described in this chapter, are individuals with their own histories, at various stages of their struggle with cancer. For artists with cancer, a major motivation for making art is to cope with the associated anxiety, pain and social isolation. The work was personal, but exhibiting it in a public setting was a request to be recognized, understood and responded to. The artists' decision to show their work is an investment of trust.

In constructing one's own story via art making and then selecting work for exhibition, an artist with cancer can understand something about themselves, releasing themselves from painful experiences, evolving personally and affecting the world. They create a legacy. By communicating with others, the artists can grow as people as well. This kind of storytelling via art gives meaning to pain and can transform a life experience. It can give the artist the ability to see beyond the present or the past and it can inspire compassion. Cancer patients can pass on information and wisdom through their art which can give them a sense of expertise and reassure them their experiences are worth sharing. Exhibiting their work, they may discover their images can exert power over others as much as over themselves.

While artists have spoken eloquently about their experience of making and exhibiting art about cancer, understanding the process of synthesis and understanding undertaken by the audience involves looking at the work from the opposite angle. The power of art to provoke empathy is perhaps its most fundamental trait, tracing back to the beginning of human mark making. In fact, our brains are wired for the senses, especially vision and touch, either alone or in combination, to activate the emotional systems of the brain responsible for mirroring and sympathy. Touch need not be physically tactile, but can be elicited by seeing texture in an artwork. Whether we view a work of contemporary art or a cave painting, cells in our brain activate mechanisms for inference that include the ability to seek cause, categorize, create meaning and assign value to the images we see. Innervating our memories and past experiences of art, our empathetic brain supplies the context to connect the artwork to our own personal experiences, though an artwork need not be a "realistic" image to spark this associative recall.

Contemporary artists have addressed the subject of empathy in choreographed attempts to connect viscerally with audiences, often with tragicomic effect, as in the works of Tony Oursler, who placed round boulder-shaped sculptures under furniture and projected pleading videos of human faces, eyeballs or simply mouths asking us for help on them, all to examine the necessary conditions for empathy. Sculptor Victoria May cites the creation of empathy as a key objective of her abstract, two- and three-legged sculptures that assume poses associated with slinky models or defiant adolescents. The artist Mike Kelley, who ultimately committed suicide, sought refuge from the isolation of his depression with works that included artifacts of the loss of his dying cat, quilts made of cast-off hand-crocheted afghans and dejected stuffed animals. It appears that references to the human figure are the most direct route to eliciting empathy as are narrative works of art, although even the most abstract work can provoke powerful associations, memories and feelings.

In January 2017, art professor John Seed of Mt. San Jacinto College in Southern California sent out a Facebook inquiry asking artists: "What is the role of empathy in your art?" A few of the responses serve as an overview of the collective whole:

> Making art assumes empathy. Making art is an act of sharing. It is by definition, an invitation to others to leave their isolation and meet others on the same road as you.
>
> —Steven Holmes

> Empathy is key as it speaks the language of connection, i.e. connection to the life experiences of the viewer. We are all connected in pain, joy, fear, wonder, hunger, yearning... all we experience. Empathy in art banishes isolation and invites healing.
>
> —Nancy Good

> Most of my work stems from an emotionally charged, at times dark, at times painful place. To hear others regard it as beautiful or meaningful to their lives is the biggest compliment. The gift is in sharing and understanding the feelings and experiences of another.
>
> —Franck De Las Mercedes

> Without empathy art becomes a technical exercise.
>
> —Dab Zabooty

> Artists are the voice of the people; empathy is what is channeled by many artists to express what needs to be seen or heard from the public when the world is in confusion.
>
> —Joao de Brito

> Empathy is essential for discerning truth
>
> —Ingrid Reeve (2017)

When viewing the work of art by people with cancer or cancer survivors, we are accepting their invitation to look at the world from another's perspective, to be empathetic. Walking through the exhibition "From the Canvas to the Couch: Art and Cancer" and viewing it as a sum of its parts was quite like walking into the forbidding enchanted forest of a Grimm Brothers' tale. We are invited into a world of knives and blood, rotten cupcake-like breasts, dark, bloodred landscapes, illustrated stories of depression and loss and a recreation of the altered reality caused by a brain tumor. Zizi Raymond's performative diary of the remains of food she ate recalls the deprivation and overfeeding of Hansel and Gretel, where sweets become enticements to enter a nightmare, and Raymond's photo of a pear core conjure images of Sleeping Beauty's poisoned apple, despite the real progress that Zizi was making toward learning to eat again after a serious surgery. The art is unnerving, especially after you invest time looking at it and understanding its meaning. Empathy is not an anodyne or touchy-feely concept when it comes to what these artists have been experiencing.

> When we stand in front of a picture or a sculpture the boundaries of the subjective and the cultural are being negotiated. Our inner experience, when we face an emotionally moving art piece changes, as we project out own personal and cultural norms onto these images while mediating the personal- psychological with the cultural, public narrative. The viewer might have a strong affective response as we might identify with the loss portrayed in the art that goes beyond empathy, as it might pierce through our own personal memory archive. Looking at art created by artists who have cancer might actually help the viewer working through their own memory work after loss
>
> (Dreifuss-Kattan, 2017)

Works of art are bland objects until we begin to carefully perceive and interpret them. Artwork is always about something. Art requires active engagement, and it is through our interpretation of art that we make it meaningful. Art made by artists of cancer require an understanding on the part of the viewer: no single interpretation of the artwork exhausts the meaning of the art, but neither is the interpretation limited by the artist's statement or intention, or indeed stage of illness. The messages aren't always apparent in the typical 30-second gallery look. Audience members can start interpreting by making their own survey of the work. A viewer can begin by examining the work's media (the material from which an artwork is made and the techniques used on those materials), its form (how the work is composed and uses line, texture, color, scale and space), its context (the year it was made and the circumstances that surround its making) and its content (which includes subject matter and cultural reference). Following the completion of this inventory, they can take the essential next step, the move from descriptive facts to the conclusions facts provoke. Emotional reactions serve as a key to this step of interpretation. Feelings emerge which must be articulated and understood not as an end, but as a means of discovering what to ask next. Interpretation requires an understanding of what we see in the artwork that triggers an emotion, as much as the artwork's characteristics themselves.

Art educators have attempted to answer the question of what makes a good interpretation. One theory is that good interpretations provide

answers to the questions that an individual poses in response to the artwork. A satisfactory viewing experience is provided when the viewer can
answer their own questions by relating what one sees in the artwork to
one's own experience. A great experience with art, by contrast, leaves
one with a basis for thinking about the work after one leaves the exhibition space. Taking the time to create a satisfying interpretive experience allows one to gain knowledge about a particular artwork and about
oneself. When people share and compare their interpretations with each
other, the level of understanding can grow exponentially because not
everyone notices the same thing when they view art. Interpretations can
vary widely.

Yet we should not pass too quickly over the point that as these artists
distill the individual stories they wish to tell, they must fight for space
among alternative, and perhaps fictitious, representations of themselves.
As an audience, we must ask ourselves where we learn what we think we
know about cancer. How much are our concepts of cancer shaped by popular movies like *The Fault in Our Stars, 50/50, Terms of Endearment* and
the buddy film *The Bucket List*, for example, where attractive movie stars
lose their hair but keep their eyebrows and eyelashes; where patients die
without suffering and others find love, sometimes even in their cancer support group, and always have great sex? Or by television commercials that
show smiling patients meeting with distinguished and friendly doctors?
Our ideas about doctors and patients, the dying and the caretakers have
been shaped by years of exposure to actors playing roles, most often to sell
us a product or service. There is no reality where television patients play
with children in brightly lit kitchens while in the background a disembodied voice reads off a long list of vile side effects that seem to have nothing
to do with these active and healthy-looking adults. The news media shows
cancer through the lens of statistics and medical breakthroughs, health
scandals and economic arguments about insurance coverage, yet cancer
itself is absent.

To interpret the "cancer" artwork, we will, first, need to compare what
we see with what we viscerally experience when looking at the work, and,
then, we must associate those factors with, or distinguish them from, our
experiences outside of the art gallery. Viewing the art production of cancer
survivors may require us to give up some of our preconceived ideas and to
re-evaluate our common sense, or our illusions.

Studies have demonstrated that exhibition visitors naturally use and appreciate galleries and museums for the experience of introspection. Lois
Silverman defines introspection as a process that involves identifying, reflecting upon and understanding one's feelings, experiences and thoughts
(Silverman, 2010, pp. 45–47). Introspection is an important tool in personal
growth. For people coping with cancer, as well as their families and friends,
introspection is an essential step toward empathy. Moreover, Silverman

points out that exhibitions are important tools for raising public awareness of the social dimensions of key health issues.

We can deduce that audience members with cancer, as well as family and friends of cancer patients, bring very specific identity-related needs to the exhibition space: whether to learn more about the experience of loved ones or to validate their own feelings about the experience of cancer. Yet it is not only these groups that maintain some kind of identity-based relationship to the disease: indeed, few individuals in the United States today have not been screened for cancer, or somehow initiated into its associated mystery and fear. As they witness women and men with cancer meeting this anxiety and loss with creativity, the everyday cancer-free viewer relieves some of his or her own anxieties and comes face to face with its human portraits. In my own case, working with the artists that exhibited in "From the Canvas to the Couch" taught me that life, in short, just goes on in spite of cancer: sick parents still have to cope with problems at work or with raising children despite its debilitating effects.

Most intriguing, however, are the revelations cancer art can provoke in caretakers. In the early 1990s, Canadian artist Robert Pope began a series of realistic paintings about his experience with doctors and hospitals after he was diagnosed with Hodgkin's disease. Over the course of a decade, Pope visited and sketched radiology labs, children's hospitals, chapels and day clinics and accompanied doctors on their rounds. After consulting with therapists, ministers and nurses and showing his work to his own cancer doctor, Pope created a book and traveling exhibition that was shared with medical personnel, intended to immerse them in the patient's perspective and to emphasize the importance for holistic care. Medical students in particular were struck by how different the view of the hospital room was from the patient's eye: they had never detected patients' fear, lack of faith in treatments, isolation and the disruption of their lives. Pope concluded that cancer is unlike heart disease, or other fatal illnesses, because it is synonymous with death and fear; the physically healthy public's common response to it is avoidance or to treat it as taboo. Pope tells us that isolation is a particularly acute and compounding effect of a cancer diagnosis, to which art can provide an expressive antidote. But it can also lessen isolation for others as it might catalyze changes in therapeutic methods.

Exhibits like "From the Canvas to the Couch" remind us that if cancer is a stigma which causes the cancer-free public to fear, reject and avoid the issue of illness and loss, then it is through our openness to its individual stories that we might overcome our avoidance and break down the otherness that cancer inflicts upon its human hosts. One suggestion to exhibition organizers who take on projects like this one would be to encourage visitors to respond to questions like: "What is the emotional impact of this exhibition for you?" or "How do you see cancer differently after viewing this exhibition?" An activity that allows the audience to respond would teach curators, health workers and therapists important information about how "outsiders" respond to the work and would encourage the audience to become more mindful of their own reactions.

Moreover, opportunities beyond the exhibition itself to guide people through their interpretations of it would be very valuable. Exhibitions about the experience of cancer are disturbing. They confront the viewer with the unbending truth about surgery, illness, trauma, death and dying. Art talks with the artists, question and answer periods and workshops associated with these exhibitions can open a space for informed interpretation, as well as promoting awareness and offering opportunities for the artists and other cancer survivors to overcome isolation. In these interactions, viewer, patient and artist would all gain the possibility of empathetic contact, together realizing what makes us human and coming to a safer relation to fears they could not mitigate alone.

References

Barrett, T. (2003). *Interpreting Art: Reflecting, Wondering, and Responding.* Boston, MA: McGraw-Hill.

Carr, C. (2012, June 18). *David Wojnarowicz.* Interview. Retrieved from www.interviewmagazine.com/art/david-wojnarowicz#_.

Derrick, L. (2017, June 20). *Lavialle Campbell: Quilting in the Shadows.* The Huffington Post. Retrieved from www.huffingtonpost.com/entry/lavialle-campbell-quilting-in-the-shadows_us_594965d5e4b0579a1f392743.

Dreifuss-Kattan, E., Carey, C., Lightweaver, C., Meyers-Turner, A. Raymond, Z., & Walter, M.E. (2013). *From Cancer to the Couch: Art and Cancer.*

Dreifuss-Kattan, E. (July 2017). Personal Communication.

Falk, J.H. (2016). *Identity and the Museum Visitor Experience.* London: Routledge, Taylor & Francis Group.

Frank, P. (2016, June 21). *Diagnosed with Rare Terminal Cancer, Artist Finds Acceptance through Art.* Arts & Culture. Retrieved from www.huffingtonpost.com/entry/diagnosed-with-a-rare-terminal-cancer-artist-finds-healing-and-acceptance-through-art_us_57682495e4b0fbbc8beb1bf64.

Kandel, E. R. (2016). *Reductionism in Art and Brain Science: Bridging the Two Cultures.* New York: Columbia University Press.

Kaylin Andres: VIATICUM Press Release." (2016, June 4). *Artsy.* Retrieved from www.artsy.net/show/jenn-singer-gallery-kaylin-andres-viaticum.

LAVIALLE CAMPBELL—Modern Art Blitz episode #77 part 3. [video file]. Retrieved from www.youtube.com/watch?v=DjQLWgQ0J_M.

Perreault, J. (2007, September 19). *Hannah Wilke's Farewell.* Artopia. Retrieved from www.artsjournal.com/artopia/2007/09/hannah_wilkes_farewell.html.

Pope, R. (1991). *Illness and Healing: Images of Cancer.* Nova Scotia: Robert Pope Foundation.

Rollins, T. (1993). *"Untitled" (Beginning): An Interview with Felix Gonzalez-Torres.* Retrieved from www.artpace.org/works/iair/iair_spring_1995/untitled-beginning.

Seed, J. (2017, January 16). *I Asked Artists About Empathy: Here Is What They Said....* *The Huffington Post.* Retrieved from www.huffingtonpost.com/entry/i-asked-artists-about-empathy-here-is-what-they-said_us_587bbac0e4b094e1aa9dc740.

Silverman, L. H. (2010). *The Social Work of Museums.* London: Routledge.

Stachelhaus, H. (1991). *Joseph Beuys.* New York: Abbeville Press.

Vine, R. (1994, May 31). *Review of Exhibitions: Hannah Wilke at Ronald Feldman.* Art in America. Retrieved from https://web.archive.org/web/20071128093347/http://findarticles.com:80/p/articles/mi_m1248/is_n5_v82/ai_15406252.

Scribble, cut, paste and paint

Creative transformation through artistic play at home

Esther Dreifuss-Kattan

We all like to be creative: playing or composing music, dancing or choreographing a dance, taking photographs or even making movies with our camera or cell phone. We can sit down at a table and make some drawings, draw on our iPad or phone, or stand in front of an easel and paint a picture. For all of these creative activities, however, we need to have an idea of what we are going to express and in what form. And once we come up with an idea, then we might not be sure what material we should use and what exactly we want to express.

When we are confronted with cancer or any other illness with its diagnosis, treatments, symptoms and multiple doctors and health care workers, we are often initially afraid and confused by these new circumstances. While we may talk to our partner, friends, family members, nurses or oncologist, we also value our privacy, aloneness, insightfulness and personal creativity. We might feel anxious, depressed, tired and confused, all feelings that often are not very easily shared with loved ones who have not experienced it before themselves. However, we do want to communicate it to somebody, so that our personal experiences will no longer make us anxious, depressed, confused or withdrawn. One solution to this problem it to start making art at home alone or with a friend, partner, child, mother, father or anyone else you feel good about.

The following suggestions make it a little easier to come up with an idea for a drawing, a sculpture or a painting, providing possible titles and some suggestions for a particular media to choose from. These ideas are only suggestions, but they might stimulate your unconscious or conscious fantasies and make it easier to start the process of creative expression.

Not everybody has an art therapy group to go to and not all of us are trained to be artists. But my many years of experience with working with cancer patients has taught me that we all can express ourselves creatively and the more we do it, the better artists we become. Even more importantly, once we have created a picture and look at it, we might actually learn something about ourselves in the here and now or from our past. We might realize that our depression had lifted for the day, that we enjoyed ourselves and might be amazed how fun it was to play around with colors and lines, symbols and concepts. We might feel more confused or depressed; this, however, happens very rarely and thus might be motivation to seek help from a psychooncologist, psychologist, psychoanalyst, art therapist or clinical social worker. Even then some of your pictures might be useful and can be shared in the therapeutic process.

These exercise ideas can be altered to meet your own needs. If you choose to show these art pieces to your friends, children, doctors, partner or anybody on your social media feed, realize that you might be cheered on or criticized. Don't take it too seriously; it is your own imagination, nobody else's. Or you can just put the picture, collages and paintings into your folder for your own enjoyment and as a document of this particular challenging time in your life. Enjoy playing!

Warm ups

Scribble or Squiggle. With eyes closed, make a scribble in one color. Open your eyes and fill in the rest, making a real picture out of it using different colors. Add a title. What might it be? What do you see? What can you connect it with?

Three Forms. Outline three geometric forms, and use a different color for each. Fill them with color and connect them in an attempt to make a story or an object. Could be concrete or abstract.

Speed Collage. Take one magazine and pick out three pages and cut out three images, or colors, or letters or numbers. Make a collage in ten minutes with scissors and a glue stick. Give it a tile. What comes to mind?

My Mood. Write a sentence that describes your mood at this moment. Translate this mood into a landscape with colors. Can be concrete or abstract. Use acrylic paint or watercolor.

Three Lines. Draw three different lines such as a squiggly line, a sharp line, a curly line, a zigzag line. Make your lines with three different colors with three different materials, like pencil, marker, paint, ink, magic marker or colored pencils. Give it a title.

My Collage Diary. Create a collage diary day by day for one week. Spend no more than 20 minutes in a single day. Write a story line for your diary, give it a title and make sure you include the date and year.

Colors. Choose one color. Then the opposite color. Draw a picture and come up with a title. All this in ten minutes. Are you surprised?

Graphic Dialogue. Choose a friend or a family member to make a drawing with. Each of you should use only one color. One person starts drawing while the other looks on for no longer than 30 seconds. Afterward the second person adds to the drawing of the first for 30 seconds. Go back and forth like this until the picture seems finished. In the end, talk about what you have made and both of you should come up with a title. Did your collaborator make boundaries? Were you relaxed or bored, inspired or anxious? Did a cohesive image appear?

Personal

Self-Portrait with a Hat. Make an acrylic painting on a canvas. Think of a title. Is it you? Not you? Who could it be? Why did you choose this hat?

My Ideal Self. You can depict just your face or your entire body. How would you like to look? Would you like to be younger or older? Bigger or smaller? What is your expression? What can you learn about yourself?

How Do I Feel Today? What is your dominant feeling today? Express the feeling using oil crayons. What comes to mind when you look at it? Too sunny? Too dark? Is the picture balanced?

My Favorite Fairy Tale. Illustrate a scene from your favorite fairy tale or of an important character in a fairy tale you like. Use colored paper cutouts. Explain in a paragraph why you choose it.

Family Portrait. Draw, paint or collage your family, including yourself. It can be real or as animals or plants. Give each person their name and come up with a title. Are you surprised by the size or color of the arrangement? Why? What could it mean?

Family Event. Make a painting of the best or worst event with your family when you were a child. Use pencil and watercolor. Come up with a title. What can you learn about it looking forward and then back?

My Easy and Complicated Traits. Make a collage in two parts. On one side show your good traits, and on the other side your more difficult ones, using different magazines. Can you think of a bridge between the two?

A Dialogue. Create a visual dialogue with your favorite person and then create a dialogue with your least favorite person. Use colored pencils or magic markers. What did you learn about them? Why these people and not others?

My Strength. What are you proud of about yourself? Write a free association poem (no rhyme needed) and make an illustration for it. Are you surprised?

Myself. Find a photograph of yourself and draw on it with pen and ink to alter it or free associate about it with written words and symbols on the image.

My cancer

My Oncologist. What comes to mind when you think back to when you heard your doctor tell you that you were diagnosed with cancer? Make a concrete or an abstract image of you and the doctor with two speech bubbles with the dialogue of that time. You can represent what you and the doctor actually said or what you wish you and the doctor would have said.

My Body Image. Have somebody outline your body by lying on a big piece of butcher paper. Fill it in with whatever comes to mind, starting with the feet. Is it still you?

Making Waves. Paint waves with watercolors, making them high or low, big or small, tiny or medium. Then write or collage your feelings or moods into each wave. Create a title. What do these up and downs mean?

Speak Up! Create a picture called: Speak Up! Maybe you would like to speak up to your doctor/oncologist, mother, children or supervisor. Choose any medium and color.

What is Positive about My Cancer? Think of a positive outcome of having cancer. Do you have more time now or see more friends? Are you less alone? Do you read more or speak up more...? Make a painting of the most meaningful thing, using both abstract and concrete forms.

Change? How did your relationship with your family change after cancer? Try to make a poem or song with an illustration about it. It does not have to rhyme.

My Cancer Map. Think of your cancer journey and create a map of it from diagnosis to the present. Use a strong background, cardboard, loose canvas, fabric or a Bristol paper. Draw, glue, paint and put little objects on this map till you think it is complete. It may take more than one sitting. What comes to mind?

Who Am I Besides My Cancer? Who and what are you besides your cancer? A runner, a skier, an enchanted grandmother, an inventor, a singer, a relaxed person, a child? Make a portrait of this person. Reflect on what you choose.

Pain. How do you express physical or mental pain? Make a sculpture with two different colored wires or with fabric, string and needle.

Change. How are you going to change your life after cancer now? This does not have to be realistic. Hike in the Alps, become an artist, be closer to your family, rest more, eat differently. Try to make an illustration or collage to communicate what you choose.

My Favorite Person. Who or what makes me comfortable and feel protected? My partner, a stuffed animal, my dog, my best friend? Create the object with collated cardboard and paint or make a fabric collage.

My Personal Still Life. Make a painting of a personal still life that relates to your cancer. Is it in a basket or on a plate? With what inside? Use watercolor or acrylic paint.

Thank You! Who would you like to thank and for what? Paint a picture with acrylic paint, water-soluble crayons or colored inks.

Help! Make a collage with colored paper cutouts. What help are you looking for and from whom? What form would this help take?

My New Adventure. Walking away from cancer, free associate on what you want to do next and put your energy into it. Use the medium of your choice and if needed write about it on the back. Are you amazed?

Automatic writing. Take a pen and start writing about any aspect of your cancer. Do not lift your pen, just keep writing. You can use just single words or entire sentences: they do not need to make sense. Lift your pen after ten minutes. Don't worry about spelling and such. Give it a title and reflect on it. If you wish, you can make a poem or an illustration out of it.

My Personal Flag. Use your favorite colors, symbols and patterns. You can use white or colored fabric like an old sheet, canvas or a Bristol paper. What are you advertising about yourself?

A Personal Object. Look for a personal object, like a shell, a piece of fabric or a little figurine. Make an art piece that integrates this object in some way. Think about why you chose this specific item and what comes to mind about the entire art piece.

A Nightly Dream. Illustrate a reoccurring or an especially impressive dream you had lately or in the past. Try to use multiple art materials, such as inks, pencil, fabric and markers. Then write down what comes to mind. Why did you choose this specific dream?

General

My Summers! What comes to mind when you think of "summer," either in the present or in the past? Think of one memory or wish or fantasy and make a tissue paper collage, tearing the paper and using white glue.

Postcard. Create and write a postcard to someone you know, or would like to know, from the past or present or future. Use Bristol paper and colored pencils or magic markers.

Every Day is a Masterpiece. Today what would that masterpiece be? Make a line drawing with pencil, markers or pen and ink, or combine these and write a text on a postcard.

Simple Collage. Choose one image, concrete or abstract, from a page in a magazine. Cut it out and glue it somewhere on a white piece of paper. Then choose colors, like oil crayons, inks, colored pencil or acrylic paint to continue the image expanding onto the rest of the paper in your own spirit. What did you create?

An Important Childhood Memory. Think of a childhood memory about fruit or any food and make a painting about it. Come up with a title and write a sentence about the memory.

Stressed Out! Who or what brings you comfort in time of stress? What would you like to do with that person, animal or object? Create a simple sculpture with air-drying clay or a small wood sculpture, paint it with acrylic paint and write a few sentences about it.

Together and Apart. Think about family members, friends or colleagues and create their portrait. This can be rendered abstractly, concretely or both, in any medium. Make a title. Who would that be and why?

Letters and Numbers. Choose a letter such as "A" or a number such as "7." You can only use this letter in any form or size or multiple sizes to make a composition using mixed medium. Give it a meaningful title.

Balanced? Think about your physical and/or emotional balance. Create a very simple mobile with wires or a wire hanger, hanging from it corks, and small personal objects or cutouts in fabric or paper. Give it a title. Are you amazed? Frustrated?

Illustrate Your Last Dream. Create a picture or collage of the last dream you had at night or the last one you can remember. Use any medium you feel fits the dream, such as watercolor, acrylic with inks, markers. Then take a second paper and write down all the things that come to mind. Try to free associate. Share it with your therapist or insightful friend.

My Book. Use an old book you don't need any longer and recreate and alter it. You can change the front cover, delete sentences, extract pages or change them into cutouts, hide little object inside, and make it your own and choose a title for it. Use free association, be spontaneous and take enough time, perhaps days or weeks.

My Important Relationship. Create a painting that addresses one important relationship in your life, such as mother-daughter, father-daughter, brother-sister, employee-supervisor, or you and your friend. Make a picture or comic book page communicating your issues with this person.

What Can I Change in My New Life? How would you like to change aspects of your life? Perhaps more social interaction, a different job or more time for yourself? Do you want to relax more or to change your relationship with a best friend or a parent? Use any medium you like to make a picture or several mediums and make a collage. Write a paragraph after you look at it. Why did you choose this particular subject?

My Happiest Memory of Last Week. What was the happiest thing that happened last week? Make a colored paper collage. First color two white Bristol sheets using a sponge with acrylic paint and a little water. Let them dry. On the following day create the collage by cutting pieces out of your colored paper. Put a heavy object on the collage overnight to keep it flat. Was it fun to play with your self-colored paper?

My Mood Today. Use an old newspaper and paint an abstract with only black and white acrylic. Sign it and think of a title. Did your mood change or do you feel it even more?

Inside and Outside. Find two boxes, one a medium-sized cardboard or wooden cigar box, and the other a smaller one that will fit inside the first. Decide how you would like to represent the outside, how you come across to others and how you see your inside, your moods, feelings and wishes that might not always be communicated to others. Choose your colors carefully. Make sure to use acrylic paint with not much water and wait until the surfaces are dry to continue. Realize that a box can be open or closed. Stand the box on its main surface or on its side. Boxes can be inside other boxes or have even other little objects in them. Come up with a title.

My Personal Container. Use fabric and string, thread, buttons or air-drying clay to make a purse, envelope, suitcase or pouch that can house your secrets and expectations.

Cut, Pierce and Tear! Use an unstretched canvas of the size you like. Cover it with one acrylic color, like white, black, red or purple. Let it dry, and then use different tools to alter it by tearing it, piercing it and/or cutting into it while not destroying it. Can you put it back onto a frame or hang it on a piece of wood? How did it make you feel? What came up? Create a title for it after some reflection.

My Door and My Window. Make a painting with acrylic paint or water-colors depicting a window. Then paint a second picture illustrated with a door. What can you see looking outside and looking inside? Be as creative as you can. What did you feel when you were painting these two different images? What did you learn?

My Three Favorite Items Today. Think of three random but concrete things you want or need right now. A car? A tree? Some lipstick? Make a drawing of them with colored pencils, colored inks or magic markers. Then reflect on why you need these objects right now and what they represent.

The Object of the Day. Draw an object, the first thing that comes to mind. What color would you like it to be? Add a collage with magazine images or construction paper.

Three Strangers. Look through magazines and choose three people. Put them into a scene and context, such as in a room or on the beach, dancing, resting or doing something else. Use paint to create the environment or try using only collage.

My Own Future—Next Week, Month, Year. Using fabric, string, buttons, needle and thread, make something you'd like to be or to do, a place you'd like to go, a project you'd like to accomplish, etc.

The Most Significant "Other" In My Life Right Now. Make a picture about this relationship, including yourself. Think about how and why this relationship came about, and what this relationship brings you.

My Personal Puzzle. Create a puzzle with Bristol paper and color. Choose a theme that is on your mind: nature, your bedroom or a personal space, something beautiful.

My Wish for Next Year, Month, Day! Think of something concrete, like a resolution, a person, an object or a goal. Use any medium you have ready at hand, such as pencil, colored pencils, markers or any paint to make a picture of it.

My Melody! Listen to two pieces of music and make an artwork for each. This is about free association, being in the moment, having a good time and being distracted. Use watercolor or acrylic paint to go with the musical flow. Did your mood change? What came to mind?

My Own Favorite Space. Draw a picture of where you feel most comfortable and relaxed. It might be a room in a house, in a garden or next to a pond, lake, mountain or beach. Maybe it is a yoga studio or an art studio.

Endings and Beginnings. Make an abstract painting using acrylic paint or watercolor, using the phrase "endings and beginnings" to let yourself be guided by your unconscious associations. Once you are done, write a few sentences and a title.

My Brain Map. Create a map of your personal brain, using multimedia and being as creative as you want. What do you think are the colors, forms, thoughts or feelings in there?

Worry Ball. Create a ball form leftover fabric strips, felt, strings, ribbons or any other material. Write or sew on it your main worry. Are you surprised? You can hold it or throw it. Did you gain some insight into what makes you anxious right now?

Warrior Self-Portrait. Make a self-portrait as your favorite cartoon, superhero or warrior. Use a stretched canvas and acrylic paint. What comes to mind? Are you surprised?

Index

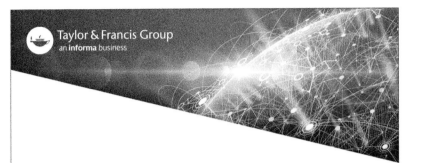